Moringa

Nature's Medicine Cabinet

Moringa

Nature's Medicine Cabinet

Sanford Holst

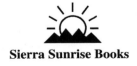

Sierra Sunrise Books

Sierra Sunrise Publishing
14622 Ventura Boulevard, # 800
Sherman Oaks, California 91403

Printed in the United States of America

First Printing: October, 2000

Publisher's Cataloging-in-Publication Data

Holst, Sanford.
    Moringa : nature's medicine cabinet / Sanford
Holst. – 1st ed.
    p. cm.
    Includes bibliographical references and index.
    ISBN: 1-887263-16-0

    1. Moringa oleifera—Therapeutic use.
2. Alternative medicine.   I. Title.

RM666.M79H65 2000   615'.321
                    QBI00-500083

Library of Congress Control Number: 00-133478

Cover photo by Gordon Daida, Aiea, HI.

Acknowledgements

I'd like to thank the wonderful people I've been privileged to work with on this adventure called Moringa.

First and foremost are Dr. Martin Price, Kristin Davis, Beth Gutheil and all the other great people at ECHO who have been instrumental in spreading the word about Moringa and inspiring projects to help people in need around the world.

Thanks also to Lowell J. Fuglie, who is actively working in Senegal to introduce Moringa to local populations most in need of nutrition and better health, as well as sharing his insights and knowledge to further spread awareness of this remarkable tree.

And to Mark Olson, whose doctoral thesis on Moringa provides excellent factual soil in which additional work can take root.

As well, to Dr. Geoff Folkard and John Sutherland at the University of Leicester in England, who have advanced not only the body of research on Moringa as a whole, but studied and documented its water-purification role to such an extent that it is now widely known and understood in scientific circles.

And last but not least, a nod to those of my stalwart friends who share the wonder of exploring this world for new ideas and bringing them to life in words...Gudrun Stutz, Sheree Noble, Larry Kurtz, Terry Gegesi, Susie Salva and Bert Crowder.

Contents

A Remarkable Discovery

*M*oringa is a remarkable discovery which can make a tremendous difference in your health and quality of life. Mounting scientific evidence shows what has been known for thousands of years by people in the tropical parts of the world: Moringa is nature's medicine cabinet.

It is best known as an excellent source of nutrition and a natural energy booster. Loaded with nutrients, vitamins and amino acids, it replenishes your body and provides what you need to get through a hectic weekday or active weekend.

As the candles multiply on top of your birthday cake, you may find yourself slowing down and saying, "I just don't feel eighteen any more." Moringa gives back some of the energy you thought was lost.

Yet this is not a sugar-based energy. It's not something which makes you hyper for some period of intense activity then leaves you drained. In fact, Moringa is also relaxing...it helps to reduce blood pressure and assure a good night's sleep. How does it contribute more energy and greater relaxation at the same time?

The answer seems to be Moringa's well documented detoxifying effect. University laboratories around the world have studied

Moringa's ability to purify water...attaching itself to harmful material and bacteria, and allowing them to be expelled as waste. The evidence points to this same process going on inside your body.

It produces long-lasting energy without hyperactivity...a nerve system at rest...a blood system not under pressure...a gland and hormone system in balance.

Other health benefits identified by people who use Moringa continue this same pattern: immune system strengthened, skin condition restored, blood pressure controlled, headaches and migraines handled, diabetes sugar level managed, inflammations and arthritis pains reduced, tumors restricted and ulcers healed.

A body that's not fighting damaging internal elements is better able to use the nutrients which come into it to build healthy skin, bone and muscles, as well as the all-important hormones which keep your body in balance.

And Moringa is loaded with nutrients. Each ounce of Moringa contains seven times the Vitamin C found in oranges, four times the Vitamin A of carrots, three times the iron of spinach, four times as much calcium as milk and three times the potassium of bananas.

One of the best attributes of Moringa is that it is also quite tasty and a welcome addition to your kitchen. The leaves, pods and flowers of this versatile tree are all edible, each with its own flavor. They can be served fresh with meals, or be reduced to powder and used as a food supplement.

That it literally "grows on trees" is an extra bonus. This wonderful tree grows outdoors in the warmer parts of the country, and can be grown indoors in other areas.

The best way to get Moringa and take advantage of its remarkable health benefits is to get seeds and grow your own. This gives you an unlimited supply, fresh every day. I'll show you where to get the seeds and how to raise vibrant, productive plants.

But if you want to try Moringa right away to see what it's like and experience some of its benefits, there are also specialty markets which carry it. Almost any market which sells food from India or Sri Lanka has cans or bottles of Moringa pods identified as "Drumsticks," the popular British name for them. Organic markets and health food stores in the U.S. have just begun to stock Moringa, since its exceptional benefits have only recently been discovered here. But it's catching on quickly.

That's because Moringa's effect on people's health has been nothing short of miraculous. I'll tell you some of those stories and introduce a number of wonderful people around the world who have discovered its remarkable properties. Many of them are now working to spread the word about Moringa, especially among developing countries where its gifts are, in many cases, the gift of life.

I was already gathering information on Moringa when I read an eye-catching front page article in the Los Angeles Times. It was written by Mark Fritz, a gifted writer and budding sleuth. His story encapsulated the extraordinary benefits of Moringa and started a stampede of interest which overwhelmed tree nurseries and seed-supply shops. Moringa trees were almost impossible to find anywhere in the United States.

For many years I've been living a healthy life, exploring the new frontiers of well-being, and writing about those discoveries. When I stumbled across mention of Moringa on the Internet, it stood out like water in the desert. And like that water, it gave rise to so many good things that it seemed unbelievable.

What tipped the scales for me were the excellent people and organizations working to bring Moringa's benefits to other people in the world—especially where malnutrition and health problems are so severe that Moringa is literally the difference between life and death. Nonprofit organizations, religious groups and university researchers are dedicated to this effort...convinced by the scientific evidence of its benefits. My research has confirmed what they found, and you'll see ample evidence of it here.

Moringa has another, very personal, aspect to it also. I grow it at home and, living in Southern California, have planted it outdoors as well. There is something special about being able to harvest the tender green leaves and put them directly into your salad.... Or pick the green pods, which are very much like large string beans, and eat them as part of dinner a few minutes later... Or take a handful of the fragrant flowers to make a cup of aromatic, soothing tea. Moringa becomes a positive part of your life with very little effort.

In terms of where it came from, the Moringa tree is native to Northern India. It was well-known to ancient Sanskrit writers as a medicinal plant. In Ayurveda, which records the Hindu art of medicine and life, it is said the leaves of the Moringa tree prevent 300 diseases.

Ancient Roman, Greek and Egyptian civilizations used the pleasant-tasting edible oil extracted from Moringa seeds for making perfume and protecting their skin.

For thousands of years, this amazing tree has slowly spread to other tropical lands, going west to the Horn of Africa and east to the Philippines. Today, its seeds have been carried by hand to country after country around the world.

Although Moringa is the universal name for this tree, it's also known as the Drumstick tree (U.K.), Horseradish tree (U.S.), Ben aile (France), Sajna (India), Murunkak-kai (Sri Lanka), Malunggay (Philippines), Mlonge (Kenya), Nebeday (Senegal) and Benzolive (Haiti).

By any name it is—to many—the gift of better health and a better life.

Medicinal Properties

Moringa is one of the most powerful health-enhancing plants that has ever been discovered. While many things found in Nature can have a remarkable effect in one or two areas, Moringa is outstanding in so many different ways.

Over the years, I've enjoyed participating in a number of breakthrough discoveries which have had a positive effect on health. But few of them have ever been as well documented by highly reputable organizations as Moringa. In discussing the medicinal properties which make this plant special, I'll mention a number of sources. You'll find many more references in the back of this book.

If you're as intrigued by what you find as I was, each new piece will be a rewarding discovery.

Nutrition and Energy Boost

While many people with average health find that Moringa gives them a welcome boost of energy, the clearest examples of its effect on the body are seen when we consider what happens with people in poorer health.

In parts of Senegal, Moringa is given by local hospitals to people with serious health problems. When 22-year-old Maïssata prematurely gave birth to Awa, the baby weighed only 3.3 pounds. No one expected the child to live, not even her mother.

"I had no hope for my baby's life," said Maïssata. "She was so thin! And I was having problems myself. I was very weak and suffering from dizziness, and I was not producing enough milk for my baby."

She was given a bag of Moringa powder and instructed how to use it. "I began adding leaf powder to my food. A couple times I even put some powder in the formula for my baby."

Five months after her birth, Awa was a healthy 11 pound baby. And Maïssata knows why.

"It was the Moringa! After I started eating it, my dizziness went away, and I started producing enough milk. I felt healthier, and both the baby and I began gaining weight."

Moringa had saved Awa's life.

This experience, and others like it, were documented by Lowell Fuglie in 1999.[1]

Detoxification

In vitro studies have shown Moringa's ability to remove hazardous materials from aqueous solutions. Its usefulness in water purification has been demonstrated many times in University studies, in laboratories and in the field. This is widely studied because it's estimated that 1.3 billion people in the world today use contaminated water for drinking and cooking. Over 6 million children are believed to die each year from infections caused by unclean water.

G. Folkard and J. Sutherland have documented in detail the use of crushed Moringa seeds to clarify dangerously impure water.

They've reported the results of their research in Agroforestry Today[2] and many other publications.

This is also seen in the work of R. Holmes and others, who published their findings in the proceedings of the international conference "Science and Technology in Third World Development" at the University of Strathclyde in Scotland.[3]

Antibiotic

Moringa's ability to work as a gentle, natural antibiotic demonstrates the old adage that "an ounce of prevention is worth a pound of cure." If you have a raging infection, I'm fairly sure Moringa is not going to stop it. But when infections are in their early stages or are only skin-deep, it seems remarkably effective.

The first mention I found of the antibiotic properties of Moringa seeds was reported in 1981 in the Journal of Medicinal Plant Research.[4]

This antibiotic was then identified in 1983 by James A. Duke as Pterygospermin, a bactericidal and fungicidal compound.[5] Mark Olson gives the chemical description of the antibiotic compound as the glucosinolate 4 alpha-L-rhamnosyloxy benzyl isothiocyanate.[6]

A study in 1990 showed fresh Moringa leaf juice produced inhibition of the bacterium Pseudononas aeruginosa.[7] The following year an *in vitro* study showed an aqueous extract made from seeds was equally as effective against the skin-infecting bacteria Staphylococcus aureus as the antibiotic Neomycin.[8]

Skin Treatment

I've seen many references to a poultice being made using Moringa which has great healing benefits for the skin. This seems to cure cuts, scrapes, sores and rashes, as well as cracking and other signs of aging. From personal experience I can tell you it seems to work. This is discussed further in the chapter on How to Prepare and Use Moringa.

Anti-Inflammatory

The oral tradition handed down in India has long praised Moringa as an anti-inflammatory for use in healing wounds. This effect was documented in 1994.[9]

In a separate study, an extract from dried roots was applied to laboratory mice, and demonstrated clearly that the roots possess anti-inflammatory properties. An interesting side note was included: one of the researchers watched an herbalist apply freshly ground Moringa roots on what appeared to be a large, trauma-initiated chronic inflammatory swelling of the ankle. Overnight, the swelling was dramatically reduced.[10]

In another study, an infusion of seeds, roots and flowers significantly inhibited the formation of pedal edema (swelling of tissues in the foot), although the authors concluded that the seed infusion may be the only one worthy of further investigation.[11]

Immune Defense System

The ability of lectin taken from the Moringa pod to modulate the body's defense system was studied in 1994 by K.K. Jayavard-hanan and others, and published in the Journal of Experimental Clinical Cancer Research.[12]

Later field tests in Senegal verified this result, with significantly fewer illnesses occurring in villages where the use of Moringa was introduced.[1]

Ulcers

The anti-ulcer effect of Moringa was reported in 1995 in the journal Phytotherapy Research. An extract taken from dried leaves showed an impressive ability to heal ulcers in laboratory animals. Administration of daily doses by injection caused a very significant improvement in the healing rate in induced gastric ulcers.[13]

Blood Pressure

James A. Duke[2] showed in 1983 that the Moringa root-bark contained an alkaloid called moringinine which acted as a cardiac stimulant and produced an increase in blood pressure. Recipes which use the root of this tree normally recommend stripping away the root-bark first. Even so, these recipes are for a condiment which tastes like horseradish—and it could well be that this stimulant gives the seasoning its "kick." People who have high blood pressure conditions would probably be well-advised to not try recipes involving the roots of this tree.

In 1994, a team of researchers were able to isolate and identify the structure of the new nitrile and mustard oil glycosides in Moringa and study their effect on blood pressure.[14]

The following year, an aqueous extract from stem bark was shown to increase the rate of heart contractions at low concentrations and decrease the rate at high concentrations, with the effect of lowering blood pressure.[15]

Diabetes

An extract from the Moringa leaf has been shown to be effective in lowering blood sugar levels within a space of 3 hours, though less effectively than the standard hypoglycemic drug, glibenclamide. The effects increased with larger doses, as shown by E. Makonnen and others.[16]

Relaxation and Sleep

An extract made from dried, powdered leaves has been demonstrated to have a very potent depressive effect on the central nervous system, resulting in significant muscle relaxation, decreased body temperatures and increased sleep time among laboratory mice. Subjects receiving the highest dosages spent twice as much time asleep as the control group.[17]

Other Properties

An infusion made from seeds demonstrated an ability to inhibit intestinal spasms, as well as producing some diuretic activity (increased urine flow). This study was published in the Journal of Ethnopharmacology.[11]

Traditional practices by villagers who have used Moringa for many years also attest to its value in controlling spasms and as a diuretic.

An extract from Moringa leaves was found to be effective at inhibiting the growth of the fungi Basidiobolus haptosporus and B. ranarum. The *in vitro* anti-fungal effects of the extract compared favorably with effects of some conventional drugs used to treat zygomycotic infections.[18]

Moringinine, from root bark, acts on the sympathetic nervous system and acts as a cardiac stimulant, relaxes bronchioles (bronchial tube inflammation) and inhibits involuntary intestinal tract movement. Anthonine, also found in root bark, is highly toxic to the cholera bacterium, per F. Booth and G. Wickens.[19]

Spirochin, found in the roots, is anti-gram+ bacteria, analgesic, antipyretic, affects the circulatory system (by raising or lowering heart beat, depending on dose), and affects the nervous system. In high doses it can paralyze the vagus nerve. Also found in roots and seeds, benzylisothiocyanate (which works against fungi and bacteria) may be even better than medicinally utilized benzylisothiocyanate and other isothiocyanates. Reported in the journal HortScience.[20]

Traditional Treatments

Lowell Fuglie has worked with Moringa in the field for many years, and over that time has gathered many of the tried-and-true treatments used by local peoples. The laboratory research reported above has verified a number of these treatments.

In addition, he knows people who have eaten and used Moringa for years and reports, "To date, absolutely no negative side effects to even daily consumption of Moringa have been recorded."

Leaves

✠ In India, juice from the leaves is believed to have a stabilizing effect on **blood pressure** and is used to treat anxiety. In Senegal, an infusion of leaf juice is believed to control glucose levels in cases of **diabetes**.

✠ Mixed with honey and followed by a drink of coconut milk 2 or 3 times a day, leaves are used as a remedy for **diarrhea, dysentery and colitis** (inflammation of the colon).

✠ Leaf juice, sometimes with carrot juice added, is used as a **diuretic** (to increase urine flow). Eating leaves is recommended in cases of **gonorrhea** on account of the diuretic action.

- In India and Nicaragua, leaves and young buds are rubbed on the temple for **headache**.
- In the Philippines and India, a poultice made from fresh leaves is applied to reduce **glandular swelling**.
- Leaf juice is sometimes used as a **skin antiseptic**.
- In India, leaves are used to treat **fevers, bronchitis, eye and ear infections, scurvy and catarrh** (inflammation of mucus membrane).
- Leaves are considered to be **anthelmintic** (able to kill intestinal worms).
- Leaves are used as an **irritant** and as a **purgative**.
- In Nicaragua, Guatemala and Senegal, leaves are applied as poultice on **sores and skin infections**.
- In the Philippines, eating leaves is believed to increase a woman's **milk production** and is sometimes prescribed for **anemia**.

Flowers

- The flowers are traditionally used as a **tonic, diuretic, and abortifacient**. [**Caution**: for this reason, the flowers and derivatives of the flowers should not be used by women in the course of a healthy pregnancy.]
- Flowers are considered to be **anthelmintic**.

✠ They are used to cure **inflammations, muscle diseases, tumors and enlargement of the spleen**.

✠ In India, juice pressed from flowers is said to alleviate **sore throat and catarrh**.

✠ In Puerto Rico, an infusion of wet flowers is used as an **eyewash** and a decoction from the flowers has been used to treat **hysteria**.

Pods

✠ The pods are believed to be **anthelmintic**.

✠ Pods are used in affections of the liver and spleen, and in treating **articular pains** (pain in the joints).

Roots

[**Caution:** for the reasons discussed above, medicinal treatments using the roots are not recommended for people with high blood pressure.]

✠ In India, the roots are used as a **carminative** (promotes gas expulsion from the alimentary canal, against intestinal pain or spasms) and as a **laxative**.

✠ Roots are considered useful against **intermittent fevers** and are sometimes chewed to relieve **cold symptoms**.

✠ Juice from roots is applied externally as a **rubefacient** (skin tonic), **counterirritant** or **vesicant** (agent to induce blistering).

- Roots are used as an **abortifacient, diuretic** as well as a **cardiac and circulatory tonic**.

- Roots are used to treat **epilepsy, nervous debility and hysteria**.

- In Senegal and India, roots are pounded and mixed with salt to make a poultice for treating **rheumatism** and **articular pains**. In Senegal, this poultice is also used to relieve **lower back or kidney pain**.

- Roots are used as a **purgative**.

- In India, Indo-China, Nicaragua and Nigeria, a root poultice is used to treat **inflammations**, especially **pedal edema** (swelling of tissues in the foot).

- A decoction of roots is used to cleanse **sores** and **ulcers**.

- In India and Indo-China, roots are used to treat cases of **scurvy**.

- Root juice mixed with milk is considered useful against **hiccoughs, asthma, gout, lumbago, rheumatism, enlarged spleen or liver, internal and deep-seated inflammations**, and **calculous affections** (mineral build-up/kidney stones). Crushed root mixed with rum has been used as a liniment on **rheumatism**.

- A snuff made from roots is inhaled to relieve **earache** and **toothache**.

- A juice made from a combination of fresh roots, bark and leaves is inserted into the nostrils to arouse a patient from **coma** or **stupor**.

Root Bark and Stem Bark

❊ In Senegal, the root and tree bark are used to treat **sores** and **skin infections**.

❊ The bark is regarded as useful in treating **scurvy**.

❊ In India, stem and root bark are taken as appetizers and **digestives**.

❊ In Senegal, a decoction of root bark, roots, leaves and flowers is used to treat **epilepsy, hysteria, and intestinal spasms**.

❊ In India, a decoction of the root bark is used as a fermentation to relieve **intestinal spasm** and is considered useful in **calculous affections**.

❊ Stem bark is used to cure **eye diseases**.

❊ In India, stem and root bark are believed to be **aphrodisiacs** and **anthelmintic**.

❊ In India, root bark is said to prevent **enlargement of the spleen** and formation of **tuberculous glands** of the neck, to destroy **tumors** and to heal **ulcers**.

❊ Juice from root bark is put into the ear to relieve **earaches** and also placed in a **toothache** cavity as a pain killer.

❊ Bark is used as a treatment for **delirious** patients.

❊ In the Philippines, it is believed that roots, chewed and applied to a **snakebite**, will keep the poison from spreading.

❊ Bark is used as a **rubefacient** and as a **vesicant**.

✠   In India, bark is sometimes mixed with peppercorns and used as an **abortifacient** (although often with fatal consequences).

Gum

✠   The tree gum, mixed with sesame oil, is used to relieve **headaches**. This is also poured into ears for the relief of **earaches**.

✠   In Java, gum is given for **intestinal complaints**.

✠   In India, gum is used for **dental caries**.

✠   Gum is considered to be a **diuretic**.

✠   In India and in Senegal, gum is considered useful in treating **fevers, dysentery** and **asthma**.

✠   Gum is used as an **astringent** and **rubefacient**.

✠   In India, gum is sometimes used as an **abortifacient**.

✠   In India, gum is used to treat **syphilis** and **rheumatism**.

Seeds

✠   The seeds are used against **fevers**.

✠   Flowers, leaves and roots are used as remedies for **various tumors**, and the seed for **abdominal tumors**.

✠   In Aruba, a paste of crushed seeds is spread on **warts**.

⬕ In India, seed oil is applied externally to relieve pain and swelling in case of **gout** or **rheumatism**, and to treat **skin diseases**.

⬕ Seed oil is used to treat **hysteria** and **scurvy**.

⬕ Oil from the seed is applied to treat **prostate** and **bladder troubles**.

⬕ Oil from the seed is considered to be a **tonic** and a **purgative**.

References

[1] Fuglie, L.J. The Miracle Tree: *Moringa oleifera*, Natural Nutrition for the Tropics. Church World Service. Dakar, Senegal. 1999

[2] Folkard, G.K. and J.P. Sutherland. *"Moringa oleifera*: a tree and a litany of potential". Agroforestry Today. 8(3) pp. 5-8. 1996

[3] Holmes, R.G.H., V.E. Travis, J.P. Sutherland and G.K. Folkard. "The use of natural coagulants to treat wastewater for agricultural re-use in developing countries". Paper presented at International Conference "Science and Technology in Third World Development", University of Strathclyde in April 1993. pp 39-47. Glasgow. 1993

[4] Eilert, U., B. Wolters and A. Nahrstedt. "The antibiotic principle of seeds of *Moringa oleifera* and *Moringa stenopetala*". Journal of Medicinal Plant Research. 42, pp 55-61. 1981

[5] Duke, J.A. Handbook of Energy Corps. (Unpublished document). 1983

[6] http://hoya.mobot.org/gradstudents/olson/moringahome.html

[7] Càceres, A., O. Cabrera, O. Morales, P. Mollinedo and P. Mendia. "Pharmacological properties of *Moringa oleifera*. 1: Pre-

liminary screening for antimicrobial activity". Journal of Ethno-pharmacology. 33, pp. 213-216. 1990

[8] Càceres, A. "Pharmacological properties of *Moringa oleifera*. 3: Effect of seed extracts in the treatment of experimental pyder-mia". Fitoterapia. LXII(5), pp. 449-450. 1991

[9] Udupa, S.L., A.L. Udupa and D.R. Kulkarni. "Studies on the anti-inflammatory and wound healing properties of *Moringa oleifera* and *Aegle marmelos*". Fitoterapia. 65(2), pp 119-123. 1994

[10] Ezeamuzie, I.C., A.W. Ambadederomo, F.O. Shode and S.C. Ekwebelem. "Anti-inflammatory effects of *Moringa oleifera* root extract". International Journal of Pharmacognosy. 34(3), pp. 207-212. 1996

[11] Càceres, A., A. Saravia, S. Rizzo, Z. Lorena, E. DeLeon and F. Nave. "Pharmacologic properties of *Moringa oleifera*. 2: Screen-ing for antispasmodic, anti-inflammatory and diuretic activity". Journal of Ethnopharmacology. 36: pp. 233-237. 1992

[12] Jayavardhanan, K.K., K. Suresh, K.R. Panikkar and D.M. Vasudevan. "Modular potency of drumstick lectin on the host de-fense system". Journal of Experimental Clinical Cancer Re-search. 13(3), pp 205-209. 1994

[13] Pal, S.K., P.K. Mukherjee and B.P. Saha. "Studies on the antiul-cer activity of *Moringa oleifera* leaf extract on gastric ulcer mod-els in rats". Phytotherpy Research. 9, pp 463-465. 1995

[14] Faizi, S., B.S. Siddiqui, R. Saleem, S. Siddiqui and K. Aftab. "Isolation and structure elucidation of new nitrile and mustard oil glycosides from *Moringa oleifera* and their effect on blood pres-sure". Journal of Natural Products. 57(9), pp 1256-1261. 1994

[15] Limaye, D.A., A.Y. Nimbkar, R. Jain and M. Ahmad. "Cardio-vascular effects of the aqueous extract of *Moringa ptery-gosperma*". Phytotherapy Research. 9, pp. 37-40. 1995

[16] Makonnen, E., A. Hunde and G. Damecha. "Hypoglycaemic ef-fect of *Moringa stenopetala* aqueous extract in rabbits". Phyto-therapy Research. 11, pp. 147-148. 1997

[17] Pal, S.K., P.K. Mukherjee, K. Saha, M. Pal and B.P. Saha. "Studies on some psychopharmacalogical actions of *Moringa oleifera* Lam. (Moringaceae) leaf extract". Phytotherapy Research. 10, pp. 402-405. 1996

[18] Nwosu, M.O. and J.I. Okafor. "Preliminary studies of the antifungal activities of some medicinal plants against Basidiobolus and some other pathological fungi". Mycoses. 38, pp. 191-195. 1995

[19] Booth, F.E.M. and G.E. Wickens. "Non-timber uses of selected arid zone trees and shrubs in Africa". FAO Conservation Guide. pp 92-101. Rome. 1988

[20] Palada, M.C. "Moringa (*Moringa oleifera* Lam.): A versatile tree crop with horticultural potential in the subtropical United States". HortScience. 31(5). September, 1996

Helping the World's Needy

One of the great things about Moringa is the fact that it not only gives a positive boost to people of average health, but can tremendously benefit the estimated one billion people around the world who suffer from seriously poor health and malnutrition. For some, Moringa is saving lives.

The immediate benefits Moringa provides to people with serious health problems has inspired several organizations to mobilize programs. They are bringing this life-saving tree to people who truly need it.

Among the dedicated people and organizations doing this work are three who are really exceptional: Trees for Life, the Educational Concerns for Hunger Organization (ECHO), and the National Council of Churches (NCC).

The following project from the NCC and its Church World Service is an example of the work being done in Africa and Asia to help those people in the world who are most in need.

Mother and Child Health Project

All of us are indebted to people like Lowell Fuglie who share our good intentions, but who also act on them to create good deeds which directly benefit thousands of people.

Lowell arranged a program in the West African country of Senegal to combat malnutrition among infants and women of child-bearing age by using Moringa. This effort was sponsored by CWS and the local Senegalese organization AGADA. He also went a step further and documented the results of this program in his 68-page book, "The Miracle Tree *Moringa Oleifera*."

Although Moringa grows wild in Africa, the leaves were only rarely used for food. Even then, much of the nutritional content was lost by the local practice of boiling the leaves and discarding the water as many as three times before eating the leaves.

Here are some of the experiences from this two-year project in which local health care providers were trained to go out among the people and show how this tree could improve their life.

Atabou Mané, supervisor of the primary health care department at the hospital in Bignona, Senegal, participated in the program and had this to say.

"We have always had problems with the classical approach to treating malnourished children. This was based on industrial products: whole milk powder, vegetable oil and sugar. All these things are expensive. When you tell a parent to go out and buy these things—this can be truly costly for him. On the other hand, with Moringa the resource is locally available. The people themselves can produce it.

"We have done experiments in treating malnourished children with this plant and the results have been really spectacular. Now, when women bring their children to our hospital we explain to them about Moringa and show them how to prepare it.

"Personally, I often suffered from fatigue. These days, when I feel tired I will eat Moringa and afterwards I always feel much better. I believe that if we can promote this tree on a large scale we could solve many problems. This year, during the wet season, we will plant Moringa trees behind the hospital."

N'Deye Sakho, a colleague of Mr. Mané and nurse in charge of pediatrics at the hospital, pointed out, "When women bring their children here, we weigh the child and give medicines for any disease he has. Then we explain to the mothers the importance of Moringa and advise them to put a little bit of leaf powder in the child's food every day. From what we've seen so far, it is really an excellent product. When women bring back their child some time later, we hardly recognize them."

Siaka Goudiaby, an administrator at the general hospital in Ziguinchor, Senegal, needed little convincing when he was approached about spreading the word on Moringa. A diabetic, he had been controlling his blood sugar levels for three years by periodically drinking a tea he made from Moringa leaves. He reported, "We are going to plant one thousand trees this year around the hospital complex. That way we will always have a ready supply of leaves to treat the cases of malnutrition we receive."

During an eight month period the hospital treated 45 malnourished children, 20 of whom were in serious condition, adding Moringa leaf powder to infant formulas. 17 of the severely malnourished and all 25 of the moderately malnourished children enjoyed full recoveries. Sadly, the other 3 children were unable to be helped.

Souadou Sagna, like other participants in the informational programs conducted in the area, received a small sack of leaf powder to take home and try. She added two spoonfuls of powder to a palm oil sauce and had this reaction.

"My son really liked the sauce. He asked me where I had learned to make it! Since then we have had the sauce on several occasions and I have prepared the pods three times. I no longer feel the fatigue I used to suffer from all the time. Since the first day, my children and I have seen the virtue of this plant."

An important part of the program was the trips made by two trainers going from village to village, giving talks to groups of people about the nutritional value of Moringa. They not only discussed the health benefits, but demonstrated different ways to prepare the leaves and pods.

An outside evaluation of this project was conducted in December, 1998 by regional health officials. They interviewed 70 people in order to get statistically-meaningful results. This is what they found.

"Through the project's collaboration with local health posts, successful treatment of malnourished children has been well-documented. Interviews with men and women who have made Moringa a regular part of their diets point out that they have a keen awareness of improvements in their health and energy. The evaluation cited two villages where the women remarked on the general improvement in health, particularly among the children, since the Moringa promotion.

"People interviewed have expressed every intention of continuing to include Moringa in their diets because of the sense of physical well-being it gives them. The evaluation cited the village of Coubalan where virtually every household now maintains a stock of Moringa leaf powder.

"This has been surprisingly successful, since new foods are often very difficult to introduce in West Africa. People interviewed have shown considerable inventiveness when it comes to preparing Moringa pods, seeds and flowers.

"Partly through training provided in local communities...and partly through ordinary word-of-mouth and example, Moringa and its properties are gradually becoming known even outside the project's target area. The project directly sponsored the planting of 10,000 trees in 1998, but it is likely that a similar number were planted by individuals within the region."

To learn more about NCC's programs, contact:
Church World Service (CWS)
Agricultural Missions
475 Riverside Drive, Room 624
New York, NY 10115
Tel: 212-870-2553

Fax: 212-870-3220
Email: dorisr@nccusa.org
Web: www.churchworldservice.org

Trees for Life

Since Trees for Life was started in 1984, more than 2.5 million people have participated in its programs. As a result, more than 30 million trees have been planted in developing countries.

For a small donation, Trees for Life will plant 10 fruit trees in a developing country, in the name of a person you designate. Then they send a certificate to that person as an acknowledgement, reporting the trees were planted.

This organization also provides highly useful information on their website, which is frequently updated. Read more about Trees for Life there.

They can be reached at:
Trees for Life
3006 W. St. Louis
Wichita, KS 67203
Tel: 316-945-6929
Email: info@treesforlife.org
Web: www.treesforlife.org

ECHO

ECHO is a nonprofit organization dedicated to the fight against world hunger. Its Internet site not only provides information, but also allows groups around the world to access its resources and services in support of small farm tropical agriculture.

Seeds of useful plants which grow in tropical areas are provided free of charge to small farmers or urban gardeners in the third world. They also make these seeds available at a small charge to others who request them.

ECHO maintains a farm at their center in Florida which raises a wide variety of beneficial plants and demonstrates innovative agricultural techniques. Free tours of the site are available to the public.

The online technical notes provided by ECHO contain excellent information on Moringa and other useful plants. The people I've talked with there are always helpful and knowledgeable, and a delight to work with.

You can reach them at:
ECHO
17391 Durrance Road
N. Fort Meyers, FL 33917
Tel: 941-543-3246
Fax: 941-543-5317
Email: echo@echonet.org
Web: www.echonet.org

Water Purification

According to Dr. Geoff Folkard at the University of Leicester in England, about 1.3 billion people in the developing world are compelled to use contaminated water for drinking and cooking purposes. And over 6 million children are believed to die each year from infections caused by unclean water. Moringa is widely regarded by water purification experts as one of the best hopes to reduce the incidence of waterborne diseases.

In developed countries, water authorities use chemicals such as aluminum sulphate to solidify impure particles which are then removed at the water treatment works. In developing countries chemicals like this are scarce and expensive, and therefore not widely used. In stark contrast, powder made from Moringa seeds has been found to be as effective as these chemicals. Yet the

Moringa tree can be grown locally, providing a virtually unlimited source of material for water purification.

Victor Essou Fagnon of the Participatory Development Resource Centre—Africa, United Nations Volunteers, provides this simple way to purify water using Moringa.

"Collect the Moringa seeds, peel them, and grind the inner seeds into a powder. Pour the powder into the dirty water, and mix the solution with a stick for a couple of minutes. Leave the mixture to rest for a couple of hours—you will see that the mud and other dirt settles at the bottom of the container. Recover the clean water on top and leave it to stand in the sun for a few hours. With this method the rate of infection from water can be reduced by 80-98%. Recommended doses: from 30 to 200 milligrams of Moringa powder per 1 litre of water, depending on the quality of the water to be treated."

> "Then Moses led the people of Israel on from the Red Sea, and they moved out into the wilderness of Shur and were there three days without water. Arriving at Murah, they could not drink the water because it was bitter.
>
> "Then the people turned against Moses. 'Must we die of thirst?' they demanded.
>
> "Moses pleaded with the Lord to help them, and the Lord showed them a tree to throw into the water, and the water became sweet."
>
> Exodus 15:22-7

Other Uses for Moringa

In addition to using Moringa for medicine, food, and water purification, these are some of the other ways it is being used in developing worlds, according to Booth and Wickens:

Alley Cropping: With their rapid growth, long taproot, few lateral roots, minimal shade and large production of high-protein biomass, Moringa trees are well-suited for use in alley cropping systems.

Animal Forage: Leaves are readily eaten by cattle, sheep, goats, pigs and rabbits. Leaves can also be used as food for carp and other fish.

Domestic Cleaning Agent: Crushed leaves are used in some parts of Nigeria to scrub cooking utensils or to clean walls.

Dye: The wood yields a blue dye which was used in Jamaica and Senegal.

Fertilizer: The seed cake (left after squeezing the seed for its oil), although unsuitable as animal feed without treatment to remove the alkaloid and saponin content, can be used as a protein-rich plant fertilizer.

Gum: The gum produced from a cut tree trunk has been used in calico printing, in making medicines and as a bland-tasting condiment.

Honey Clarifier: Powdered seeds can be used to clarify honey without boiling. Seed powder can also be used to clarify sugar cane juice.

Honey Producer: The flowers are a good source of nectar for honey-producing bees.

Live Fencing: A common use for Moringa trees is to produce live supports for fencing around gardens.

Ornamental: In many countries, Moringa trees are planted in gardens and along avenues as ornamental trees.

Plant Disease Prevention: Incorporating Moringa leaves into the soil before planting can prevent damping-off disease (Pythium debaryanum) among seedlings.

Pulp: The soft, spongy wood makes a poor firewood, but the wood pulp is suitable for making newsprint and writing paper.

Rope-Making: The bark of the tree can be beaten into a fiber for production of ropes or mats.

Tannin: The bark and gum can be used in tanning hides.

How to Prepare
and Use Moringa

Now that you know about the health-enhancing properties of Moringa, let's look at how you can put the different parts of the Moringa tree to use.

At the present time it's very difficult to find fresh Moringa leaves, flowers and pods in our local stores. However, canned Moringa pods—called "drumsticks"—are available in almost any market carrying food from India and Sri Lanka. Typically, the canned or bottled pods in many markets are packed in brine (water and salt). When the container is opened, the brine should be poured off and the pods washed before use.

In gourmet shops you will often find the pods prepared as a curry, with ingredients such as onion, coconut milk, garlic, coriander, cummin, cinnamon, mustard, cardamom, pepper, cloves, curry leaves, dill seed, rampe, palm oil and salt. It may also be prepared as a sambar, with ingredients like plantain, brinjal, carrot, pumpkin, dhal, fennel, cummin, coriander, pepper, dry chili, saffron, palm oil, curry leaves and salt.

As mentioned earlier, Moringa is just starting to be stocked at health food stores and whole-food markets. The canned goods are already arriving, and hopefully the fresh produce will follow close

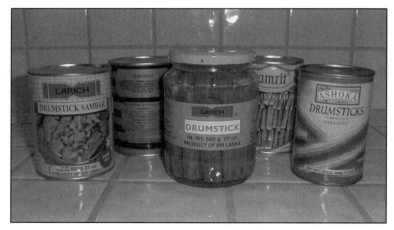

Moringa available in stores

behind. In the meantime, to get fresh leaves, pods and flowers you may have to rely on a friend who has a tree, or grow some Moringa yourself. Fortunately, growing it is a very easy process, as you'll see in the next chapter.

Right now, let's assume you have some of this wonderful bounty from Nature in your hands, and are ready to put it to good use building up your health.

Medicinal Uses

Here are some of the ways people prepare Moringa when using it for treatments. Use your discretion in deciding what course of treatment is best for you and, of course, consult your health care provider.

Since these involve leaf powder, seed powder and other useful materials made from the Moringa tree, I'll show you how to prepare those as well.

Leaf Powder

To make Moringa leaf powder, harvest some leaves from the tree. Wash them, then let them dry in an airy place out of direct sunlight (sunlight has been shown to reduce Vitamin A in this process). Rub the dried leaves over a wire screen to produce the powder. I use a food strainer made with wire mesh, which works very well for this purpose.

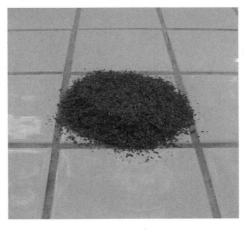

Energy Boost

This powder made from Moringa leaves seems to provide a long-lasting energy boost when Moringa is included in your diet. It works like an overall tune-up for the body, and people frequently report having much more endurance—whether in their place of work or out playing sports. This has not yet been tested to see if it benefits people with Chronic Fatigue Syndrome (CFIDS), but that seems possible.

On a regular basis, one, two or three spoonfuls of powder can be added to sauces, rice and soups just before serving (depending on the number of people being served) to provide a greater level of energy for the whole family.

I generally add a teaspoonful of the powder to a cup of fruit yogurt each morning. This works for me because my other meals are usually "on the go." The difference has been quite noticeable. Not "wired", but more stamina...especially through challenging days.

Seed Powder

Allow the Moringa pods to grow to maturity on the tree before harvesting seeds. If the harvested seeds are not completely dry, they can be sundried. Remove the shell of the dry seed to reveal the pale kernel. Then grind the kernels into powder. I use two spoons for this, grinding the kernel between the flat part of one and the edge of the other.

Ointment for Skin Treatment

As mentioned earlier, there are many reports of a poultice being made using Moringa which has great healing benefits for the skin. This seems to help cuts, scrapes, sores and rashes, as well as cracking or other signs of aging.

I have not yet found a reliable source for a Moringa ointment, but I can tell you what I use. This was developed based on research done at the University of San Carlos in Guatemala. While it is safe and effective for me, I cannot give a recommendation that you try it since it has not been used by a sufficiently large number of people to guarantee its safety.

The preparation is fairly straightforward. I place 10 grams of seed powder into 50 ml of water at 115° F for two hours, making sure the water does not boil. Then I mix one part seed-solution with 3 parts Vaseline. The resulting mixture is placed in a glass container and allowed to cool.

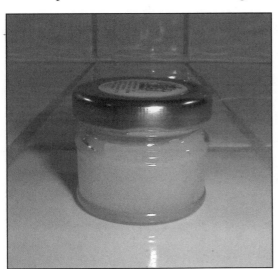

Skin ointment

The first time I used the ointment, I applied it to a very small area of skin. If there was any redness, pain or other undesired reaction, I planned to not use it. Better safe than sorry. But all went well.

Then I started using the ointment on a regular basis, applying it to the cuts and scrapes I seem to pick up as part of an active outdoor life. Trimming trees and bushes, hiking and camping tends to cause these things. When I was a little kid, these cuts healed right away. Now it takes longer. The ointment definitely seems to help. Here's the process.

I wash the area to be treated, then apply the ointment directly to the damaged skin. This is most often on the hands, arms, legs, face and neck. I'm careful not to get it in my eyes, ears or other internal area. Not because anyone said I shouldn't, but it just seems better to play it safe.

I usually repeat the treatment each evening until the problem goes away. That way I can leave it undisturbed for about 30 minutes while I read, watch television or listen to music. After that, most of it is absorbed, and I just clean off the rest with tissue paper. I don't wash the affected area at night, preferring to let the skin heal overnight.

It not only seems to heal faster, but leaves the skin feeling soft and smooth.

If a reputable company is interested in producing and testing a suitable lotion for public use, they are invited to contact me at Sandy@LifeOnNet.org.

Cold Treatment

Flowers from the Moringa tree can be used to make an aromatic tea which seems to soothe cold symptoms. The tea is made by bringing water to a boil, then dropping in a cluster of the flowers. This mixture is then allowed to steep for 5 minutes. Some people add sugar for taste, but I recommend honey instead, if available.

Herbal Remedies

Many other references cite local treatments which use Moringa leaves, flowers, pods, bark and roots for medicinal purposes, but I have not yet come across methods for how those materials are prepared and the treatments performed. I will keep looking, and may include them in future updates.

Other Treatments

One of the best "treatments" using Moringa is simply to eat it as part of your regular meals. It's quite tasty, and can be prepared in many ways. As you will see in the next section, the leaves, pods and flowers are used in a wide variety of delicious recipes.

This is probably the best way to get the detoxifying effect, strengthen your immune system, control blood pressure, heal ulcers, manage blood sugar, and all the other benefits people have identified.

Caution

Many parts of the Moringa plant have been found to be exceptionally beneficial and useful in promoting good health. However, my research into the properties and uses of this plant lead me to recommend *against* the use of the root for food.

This may seem strange, since one of the popular names for Moringa is Horseradish Tree. This name came about because Europeans in India commonly used the root as a substitute for horseradish since they are very similar in taste.

However, the root has now been shown to contain 0.105% alkaloids, especially moriginine, and a bactericide, spirochin, either of which could prove fatal when taken internally in sufficiently large quantity.

This in no way reduces the desirability of root preparations for external use.

But please take my advice and do not try recipes or internal medications involving the root at this time. Perhaps in the future there may be some medication prepared in pharmaceutical doses with specific instructions defining its use. But that day is not yet here as of this writing.

Food Preparation

The recipes shown here were gathered from all over the world. In the Philippines, people call Moringa by the name Malunggay. In addition to the recipes shown here, Filipino cookbooks can give you additional, delicious Malunggay recipes.

Some of the dishes shown here come from people who are excellent in the kitchen, but are not always painstakingly exact in their instructions. In other cases, a recipe may call for a type of fish or bean which exists only in Indonesia or Africa; if you would like to try it anyway, just substitute another type or fish or bean. As people say, "adventure is the spice of life!"

Fresh Leaves

It's easy to harvest Moringa leaves the same day you plan to use them, which guarantees they're completely fresh. Be sure to wash the leaves.

Each leaf consists of a stem with several small leaflets. Hold the stem in one hand, and slide the fingers of your other hand along it. The small, delicious leaflets literally fall into the palm of your hand.

You can also use entire Moringa seedlings or the growing tips from mature trees.

In preparing sauces, leaf powder may be used in place of fresh leaves. Cooking time can be reduced if leaf powder is left to steep in water overnight.

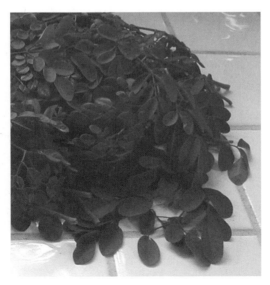

Salad

Moringa leaves are excellent in salads. They can be used as the sole source of "green," or as a flavor-enhancer and nutrition-booster when added to lettuce. Just put fresh Moringa leaves into your salad bowl, add sliced cucumbers and tomato, top with your favorite dressing, and it's ready to eat.

"Spinach"

Moringa leaves can also be prepared and used much like spinach in almost any recipe. To serve as a side dish with your meal, simply steam one cup of water with two cups of green leaflets for a few minutes until tender, mixed with butter and salt. Add other seasonings according to your taste. Serve it warm and slightly steaming at your dinner table.

Green Pods

When still very young and tender, the entire pod can be prepared and eaten in the same manner as green beans. Older pods develop a tough exterior, but their pulp and immature seeds are still edible until just before the ripening process begins. The taste of young pods is often compared to asparagus.

Kachang Kelur

In Singapore, the young pods are called Kachang Kelur, and are prepared as a dinner vegetable. The pods are scraped to remove the tough skin. The resulting, firm vegetable is then cut into pieces and boiled until soft. It is usually served warm, either just as it is, or with seasonings to suit one's taste.

Young Seeds

When the pods are not yet mature, they can be harvested and opened to reveal pale seeds inside. Often the soft pulp is also harvested along with the seeds, by scraping it out with a spoon. Wash the seeds and pulp before cooking, to remove the somewhat bitter film which coats them. The seeds at this stage look like large peas, and in fact can be prepared and used in the same way as peas in most recipes.

"Peas"

Place the young seeds (and the soft pulp, if you like) in water and bring it to a boil. Continue until the seeds are softened. Season to taste and serve while warm.

"Peanuts"

When the pods are left on the tree to grow closer to maturity, harvesting the pods and splitting them open will yield brown-colored seeds. When being prepared as food, these older seeds are usually fried on top of the stove until crispy. When allowed to cool, the seeds are said to have a peanut-like flavor.

Flowers

Flowers need to be cooked before being eaten. When fried, either alone or in a batter, they are said to have a taste similar to mushrooms. Moringa flowers may be mixed with any of the leaf recipes.

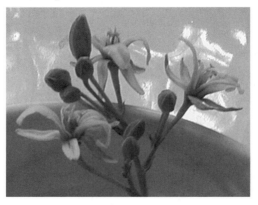

Flower Tea

Boil water, then pour it into a cup. Add Moringa flowers and allow to steep for 5 minutes. Add sugar or honey to taste. Although described previously as a cold remedy, this is also a soothing, uncaffeinated drink you can enjoy anytime.

Cooking Measures

English		Metric
1 ounce – liquid (oz)	=	29.57 milliliters (ml)
1 ounce – dry (oz)	=	28.35 grams (g)

tsp.	= teaspoon	= 1/6 ounce
T.	= tablespoon	= 1/2 ounce
c.	= cup	= 8 ounces
lb.	= pound	= 16 ounces

A booklet from Haiti written by Alicia Ray offers the following recipes. These were provided to us by the Educational Concerns for Hunger Organization (ECHO).

Haiti Vegetables

When young, the pods are edible whole, with a delicate flavor like asparagus. They can be used from the time they emerge from the flower cluster until they become too woody to snap easily. The largest ones usable in this way will probably be 12 to 15 inches long and ¼ inch in diameter. At this state they can be prepared in many ways. Here are three:

1.   Cut the pods into one-inch lengths. Add onion, butter and salt. Boil for ten minutes or until tender.

2.   Steam the pods without seasonings, then marinade in a mixture of oil, vinegar, salt, pepper, garlic and parsley.

3.   An acceptable "mock asparagus" soup can be made by boiling the cut pods with onion until tender. Add milk, thicken and season to taste.

India Peas

Ingredients:

12-15 Moringa pods
1 medium onion, diced
4 cups grated coconut
2 bouillon cubes
2 inches ginger root
4 T. oil
1 clove garlic
2 eggs, hard boiled
salt, pepper to taste

Preparation:

Blanch the peas and pulpy lining from the pods, and drain. Remove milk from 2 ½ cups grated coconut by squeezing water through it 2 or 3 times. Crush ginger root and garlic, save half for later. Mix peas, pulpy lining, coconut milk, ginger and garlic together with onion, bouillon cubes, 2 T. oil, salt and pepper. Bring to a boil and cook until the peas are soft, about 20 minutes. Fry remaining coconut until brown. Fry remaining half of crushed ginger root and garlic in 2 T. oil. Dice eggs. Add coconut, ginger, garlic and eggs to first mixture, heat through. Serves six.

The following recipes are from the Food and Nutrition Research Center, National Science Development Board (Manila) Publication No. 47, revised April 1974 and reprinted March 1978. Translation from Filipino was assisted by Earnesto Guiang, Office of Rural and Agricultural Development, USAID/Manila, and Rosalinga Garcia-Yangas, International Science and Technology Institute, Inc., Arlington, Virginia, and was provided by ECHO.

Note that coconut milk is extracted by squeezing the meat of a freshly grated coconut. The first squeezing is called kakang gata or coconut milk. A second squeezing is used after water is added to the remaining coconut meat, and this is called gata or coconut reserve.

Peccadillo with Moringa

3 c. Moringa leaves, washed
1 c. ground beef, cooked
½ c. chopped tomatoes
2 T. cooking fat
4 c. water
1 tsp. minced garlic
2 tsp. salt
1 T. sliced onion
dash of pepper

Sauté garlic, onion, and tomatoes in large fry pan. Add ground beef. Cover and simmer 5 minutes over low heat. Add water and bring to a boil. Season with slat and pepper. Add Moringa leaves. Cook 5 minutes longer. Serves 6.

Moringa Leaves Gulay

6 c. Moringa leaves, washed
1 c. coconut milk diluted with 1 c. water
1 c. dried fish (boiled, flaked and fried in 1T. cooking fat)

2 garlic cloves, minced
I medium onion, sliced
1/8 tsp. salt
4 pieces chili peppers, crushed

Boil coconut milk, dried fish, garlic and onion for 10 minutes. Season with salt, stirring mixture continuously. Add Moringa leaves and crushed chili peppers. Cook 5 minutes longer. Serve hot. Serves 6.

Shrimp Suam

2 c. Moringa leaves, washed
12 fresh shrimp, trimmed
2 T. sliced onion
2T. shortening
1½ tsp. salt
1 tsp. minced garlic
5 c. water
1 T. ginger, cut into strips
1 c. fish sauce

Sauté garlic, onion and ginger in shortening, in a large frying pan. Add fish sauce, salt and water. Bring to a boil, and add shrimp. Cover and cook 10 minutes longer. Serve at once. Serves 6.

Mung Bean Stew

3 c. Moringa leaves, washed
1 c. dried mung bean, boiled
½ c. sliced shrimp
½ c. sliced boiled pork
4 T. cooking fat
½ c. shrimp juice
1 tsp. minced garlic

½ c. pork broth
2 T. sliced onion
3 c. water
½ c. sliced tomatoes
4¼ tsp. salt
dash of pepper

Sauté garlic, onion and tomatoes in large frying pan. Add pork and shrimp. Cover and cook 3 minutes. Add mung bean, shrimp juice, pork broth and water. Cover and bring to a boil. Season with salt and pepper. Add Moringa leaves and cook 5 minutes longer. Serves 6.

Dinengdeng II

2 c. Moringa leaves
½ c. dried pigeon pea or Congo pea boiled in 1 c. water
2 large tomatoes, sliced
10 young okra, cut into 1" lengths
3 c. water
¼ c. fish paste
2 c. cowpea or yard-long bean cut into 2" lengths
½ medium onion, sliced

Add water to cooked pigeon pea or Congo pea in large saucepan. Boil, and add cowpea or yard-long bean. Cover and cook 3 minutes. Add fish paste, onion, tomatoes, fish and okra. Cover and boil 2 minutes. Do not stir vegetables. Add Moringa leaves, cover and cook 5 minutes longer. Serve hot. Serves 6.

Sautéed Moringa Pods

2 c. fresh Moringa pods
2½ c. shrimp sauce from pounded heads of shrimp
2 T. shortening
2 T. shrimp paste

1 tsp. minced garlic
1 tsp. salt
2 T. sliced onion
1 c. fresh lima or butter bean seeds, peeled
½ c. sliced tomatoes
1 c. green cowpea or yard-long bean pods cut into 1½" lengths
1 c. boiled pork, diced
½ c. shrimp, shelled and sliced lengthwise

Cut Moringa pods lengthwise into 4 pieces. Slice white pulp including tender seeds. Discard outer covering. Cut pulp into 1½" lengths. Sauté garlic, onion and tomatoes. Add pork and shrimp. Cover and cook 2 minutes. Add shrimp juice and boil. Season with fish paste and salt. Add lima or butter beans, and cook 3 minutes. Add Moringa pulp and cowpea or yard-long bean. Cover and cook 10 minutes. Serves 6.

The following list of *KPMS Recipes from the Twelve Regions* (Translation: K=pigeon or Congo pea, P=papaya, M=Moringa, S=winged bean) were compiled by Mrs. Serapia Lanuza, Home Economist Extension Specialist with the Bureau of Agricultural Extension in Quezon City, Philippines and were provided by ECHO.

Jambalaya Camp

½ c. Moringa leaves
1 c. rice
½ c. winged bean, blanched
1 onion, chopped
1 carrot, sliced thinly
3 T. oil
1 green pepper, sliced thinly
1 c. ground pork

½ c. pigeon or Congo pea seeds
¾ c. tomatoes, chopped
1 T. finely chopped celery
3 T. fish sauce
½ c. small fresh-water clams (no shell)
3 c. water (soup of boiled clams)
MSG or Accent

Wash rice and soak in small bowl for 1 hour, then drain. Fry onion in cooking oil until tender, but not brown. Set aside. Fry pork and add tomatoes and fish sauce. Add 3 c. soup of boiled clams. When boiling, stir in rice slowly on low fire. When rice is half cooked add the other ingredients. Cover tightly and cook slowly. Serve hot with sliced papaya. Serves 6.

Corn with Moringa Leaves

1 c. Moringa leaves
2 c. grated young corn
1 small sponge gourd (luffa)
2 cloves garlic
1 onion
3 c. water
Accent or MSG
Salt to taste

Sauté garlic and onion in medium frying pan. Add water and let it boil. Then add the corn, stirring often to avoid burning. When cooked, add the gourd and Moringa.

Mixed Vegetable Embotido

1 c. Moringa leaves
1½ c. pigeon or Congo peas, boiled and mashed
1 c. meat from unripe coconut
1 red pepper

1 green pepper
1 c. squash, grated
3 beaten eggs
1½ c. carrots, grated
1 onion, chopped
4 T. margarine
½ c. winged beans
1 garlic, chopped
Pepper and salt to taste

Mix all ingredients above. Wrap in plastic bags, and tie both ends. Steam for 45 minutes.

Sautéed Pigeon Pea or Congo Pea, Papaya, Moringa and Winged Bean With Liver

2 c. Moringa leaves
1¼ c. pigeon or Congo peas
½ c. liver
3 quarts water
3 T. salt
¾ c. cooking oil
2 c. water
4 segments garlic
1¾ c. winged bean
1¼ c. tomatoes

Boil peas until cooked. Set aside. Sauté garlic, onion and to-matoes. Add liver. Cover and cook until liver is tender. Season. Add water. Add winged bean and papaya. Cover and cook 10 minutes. Add cooked peas and Moringa leaves. Serve hot.

Pigeon Pea or Congo Pea with Pork and Banana Blossom

½ c. Moringa leaves
1 c. peas
1 c. winged bean
1 pc banana blossom
1 leg pork
1 c. roselle
Onions
Ginger
Salt to taste

Brown the pork. Remove from heat and cut into cubes about 2 inches in size. Boil peas and pork leg until tender. Add ginger and salt to taste. Add banana blossom and winged beans. When tender, add roselle and onions.

Chicken With Pigeon or Congo Pea, Papaya, Moringa and Winged Bean

1 c. Moringa leaves
1 medium sized chicken
1 onion
1½ c. boiled pigeon or Congo pea
1 tomato
2 pcs green medium sized Papaya
3 cloves garlic
1 c. winged beans
Salt or Accent to taste

Sauté garlic, onion and tomato. Add sliced chicken, boiled peas, and boil for 20 minutes. Then add papaya and winged beans, and boil another 10 minutes. Add Accent and salt to taste. Put in Moringa leaves before removing from heat. Serve hot.

Pigeon Pea or Congo Pea, Papaya, Moringa and Winged Bean Hamburger

½ c. Moringa leaves
1 c. boiled peas, mashed
½ c. papaya, chopped
½ c. string beans, chopped
½ c. flour
2 eggs
1 big onion, chopped
2 segments garlic
Oil to fry
Salt to taste

Sauté garlic, onions and tomatoes. Add mashed peas, papaya, winged beans, and set aside. Beat eggs and add flour. Add Moringa leaves to sautéed ingredients, and mix with beaten eggs.

Pochero A La Berding Gulay

1 c. Moringa leaves
1 c. peeled & sliced unripe papaya
3 stems green onion
1 small pc ginger (thinly sliced)
1 c. green beans or winged beans
1 T. cooking oil
3 pcs ripe tomato
5 black pepper, whole
3 pcs ripe banana
3 c. water
1 c. dried minnow
Salt to taste
1 clove garlic

Sauté the garlic and ginger in cooking oil until slightly brown. Add the water and bring to a boil. Add the banana, beans and black pepper. Cover and continue to boil. When half-done add the sliced papaya, dried minnow, tomatoes, green onions, and salt to taste. Last, add the Moringa leaves. Remove from heat when done, and serve while hot. Serves 8.

Masquadilla Torta

½ c. Moringa leaves
3 eggs, beaten
1 c. winged bean pods, finely chopped
3 pcs tomato, sliced
½ c. shredded papaya
¾ c. shredded squash
½ c. onion, sliced
½ c. powdered mung bean
5 segments garlic
¼ c. powdered dried minnow
banana leaf
Salt & pepper to taste

Mix Moringa leaves, winged bean pods, shredded papaya, squash, powdered dried minnow, powdered mung bean, tomatoes, beaten eggs, onion, garlic, salt and pepper to taste. Place one piece of 5 x 5 banana leaf on a plate, and pour the mixture on it. Then deep fry in oil until golden brown. Garnish with sliced tomatoes, onions and calamansi. Serves 8.

Pigeon or Congo Pea, Papaya, Moringa, Winged Bean Chicken Guinatan

1 c. Moringa leaves
3 pcs tomato
8 pcs winged bean
1 small papaya
1 c. coconut milk
1 c. boiled pigeon or Congo pea

1 c. palm heart
2½ c. sliced chicken
3 pcs garlic
1 small ginger
3 c. water
1 onion
Salt to taste

Sauté garlic, onions tomato and ginger in hot oil. Add the sliced chicken and boil with salt. Then add the water, and boil until the chicken is done. Add the papaya, palm heart, winged beans and pigeon or Congo pea. Last, add the Moringa leaves and coconut milk. Season to taste.

Vegetable Delight

½ c. Moringa leaves
1 c. pure coconut milk
1 small pc ginger
1/3 c. pure coconut mild reserve
3 pcs bell pepper, green & red, quartered
5 pcs fish, preferably tilapia
1 onion bulb, sliced
1-2 T. cooking oil
1 head garlic, crushed
1 tsp. crushed black pepper
3 tomatoes, quartered
½ c. pigeon or Congo peas
8-10 winged beans or string beans, quartered
1 c. cubed yellow sweet potato

Sauté garlic in oil until brown. Add onion. Transfer to un-glazed cooking pot, then add pure coconut milk, winged beans, pigeon or Congo peas, yellow sweet potato, fish and ginger. Let it boil until half-done. Add bell peppers and tomatoes. Season with salt and crushed pepper. Add the rest of the coconut milk and Moringa leaves. Boil for 5 minutes and serve.

Patalbog

 1 c. Moringa leaves
 1 c. sliced papaya
 4 c. water
 1 tsp. salt
 1 c. winged beans
 1 c. pigeon or Congo peas
 Ginger and seasoning to taste

Wash peas and papaya (which have been sliced into elongated pieces). Remove young Moringa leaves from stems. Slice winged beans to desired size and wash. Pare ginger, and pound. Place all ingredients in a casserole accordingly. Cook for 15 minutes or until all vegetables are tender. Serve hot. Serves 4.

Sautéed Young Pigeon or Congo Peas

 2 c. Moringa leaves
 2 c. dried minnow
 2 T. oil
 2 tsp. soy sauce
 1 c. young pigeon or Congo peas
 1 medium onion
 ½ c. sliced tomato
 3 cloves garlic
 1 c. sliced squash
 Salt to taste

Sauté garlic, onions and tomatoes. Add fish, squash and peas, and cover. Cook for 10 minutes. Add Moringa leaves, and continue cooking for 3 minutes. Remove from heat and serve hot.

Dinengdeng I

1 c. Moringa leaves
1 c. pigeon or Congo peas, boiled
1 T. fish paste or salted fish
1 c. green papaya, sliced into small pieces
1 pc ginger
2 medium tomatoes, sliced
1 c. winged beans, sliced into strips
1 c. roasted walking catfish or mullet

Boil 2 c. water in a casserole. Add the fish paste, ginger, and roasted fish for 15 minutes. Then add the previously boiled peas, green papaya, and winged beans. Cook until tender. Add the Moringa leaves last, and cook 2-3 minutes more. Add a pinch of Accent or salt to taste. Serve hot. Serves 4.

Pinamilit Na "Haluwan" (Dalag)

1 c. Moringa leaves
1 c. tilapia (roasted fish)
1 onion
4 c. coconut milk
1 small ginger
2 c. water
1 pc papaya
Black pepper to taste

Boil the coconut milk with water. After boiling, mix the fish with the spices for 5 minutes. Add the papaya and let it boil for 5 minutes, then add the Moringa leaves. Cook for 5 minutes more. Remove from heat. Serve hot. Serves 4.

3-In-1 Recipe

3 c. Moringa leaves
½ c. coconut milk, diluted
½ c. shrimp paste
1 c. dried shrimp
2 pcs green pepper, cut into strips
½ papaya, unripe
1 segment garlic & onion, minced

Boil coconut milk, shrimp, garlic, and onion for 10 minutes. Season with shrimp paste, and continue stirring. Add cooked peas, papaya, green pepper, and Moringa leaves. Cook 5 minutes longer. Serve hot. Serves 6.

The following recipes were provided by Lowell Fuglie, who in turn obtained them from the individuals noted at the end of this section.

The best way to prepare Moringa leaf powder for use in recipes was described earlier in this chapter, in case you would like to make some for these dishes.

While some of the recipes are not overly precise, with a little experimenting I'm sure you can make some delicious meals which appeal to your own taste.

Binga "Power" Porridge

60g maize meal
30g roasted bean meal (cowpea or any other bean can be used)
10g roasted groundnut (peanut) meal
5g sugar
Moringa leaf powder

Note that "meal" can be obtained by running the seeds through a maize mill. Finely mix the above ingredients together and prepare as you would any normal porridge.[1]

Binga "Power" Biscuits

60g maize meal
30g roasted bean meal
10g roasted groundnut (peanut) meal
20ml cooking oil
40ml water
¼ tsp. salt
½ tsp. baking powder
20g (2.5 heaped T.) Moringa leaf powder

Mix and knead all ingredients until a cohesive mass is obtained. Add more water if needed. Oil a baking tin of about 20x20cm and press the dough into the tin. (10g of roughly crushed groundnuts or sesame seeds can be pressed into the surface of the dough). Cut dough into sections using a sharp knife. Bake in a preheated oven at 170 C. for 20 minutes, or until done. Store biscuits in an airtight container.[1]

Groundnut and Millet Porridge

Millet flour
Groundnut (peanut) meal
    (use 3 parts millet flour to 1 part groundnut)
Lemon juice
Milk (fresh, powdered or condensed)
Moringa leaf powder

Mix the groundnut meal with water until a uniform paste is achieved. Put paste into a pot of boiling water (amount of water depends on whether a liquid or semi-liquid porridge is desired). Cover and boil for 15 minutes. Mix millet flour with water until a uniform paste is achieved. Slowly add this mix to the pot, stirring constantly. Cover and boil for 15-20 minutes more. Add lemon and Moringa leaf powder towards the end of the cooking process. Remove pot from fire and allow to cool, then add milk and sugar to taste.[2]

Moringa Fataya

Wheat flour
Onions
Fish (de-boned) or hamburger
Crushed red pepper
Moringa leaf powder

Mix flour with water until a dough is formed. Roll dough onto a flat surface and cut into squares. Combine onions, fish or hamburger, red pepper and leaf powder together. Put a spoonful of this sauce onto the middle of each square of dough. Fold the dough to enclose the sauce, using a fork to seal the edges. Cook in hot oil until brown.

Note: a simple doughnut can be made by mixing flour and Moringa leaf powder together, then adding water to make a dough.[3]

Moringa "Juice"

Add a spoonful or more of Moringa leaf powder to a liter of water. Add sugar to taste. Stir together. Store juice in a refrigerator.[3]

Moringa Leaf Puree

It has been reported that in the Philippines, Moringa leaves are occasionally ground into a mash, boiled and then spoon-fed to infants.[4]

Basic Moringa Leaf Sauce

2 c. fresh Moringa leaves
1 c. water
Chopped onions
Salt
Butter

Steam Moringa leaves for a few minutes in the water. Add chopped onions, salt, butter and any other seasonings according to taste.[4]

Moringa Leaf Omelet

1 bowl Moringa leaves
2 eggs
1 tsp. any bouillon soup mix
onion
tomato
garlic
salt

Wash leaves, then fry for 5 minutes with sliced onions, garlic and salt. While this cooks, lightly fry minced onion and tomatoes and add this to the fried Moringa. Stir together half a cup of this mix, two eggs, the bouillon soup mix, and cook as you would any omelet.[4]

Senegalese Leaf Sauce with Rice

Moringa leaves
palm oil
meat or fish (dried or smoked)
vegetables and spices to taste
rice

Wash leaves, then pound them into a mash using a mortar and pestle. Boil leaf mash in water until cooked (leaves turn a brownish color). Add some palm oil, meat or fish, and other desired vegetables and spices (onion, red pepper, Maggi cube). Simmer until cooked. Serve over rice.[3]

Senegalese Leaf Sauce with Millet Couscous

Moringa leaves
Groundnuts (peanuts)
Meat
Vegetables and spices to taste
Millet couscous

Wash Moringa leaves, then pound them into a mash using a mortal and pestle. Boil leaf mash in water until cooked (leaves turn a brownish color). Pound raw groundnuts into a paste, add to Moringa sauce. Add meat, vegetables and spices (onions, red pepper, Maggi cube). Simmer until cooked. Serve over millet couscous.[3]

Senegalese "Ako Nebeday" Leaf Sauce

18oz fresh Moringa leaves
18oz raw groundnut (peanut) powder
I small dried fish
5 small fresh fish or 2 pieces of any large fish
3½oz of dried fish meal
I medium onion (crushed)
1 red pepper (crushed)
3 cloves garlic (crushed)
1 Maggi cube or bouillon cube
Salt

Boil leaves, discard water, add fresh water. Add both fresh and dried fish, add salt to taste and boil again for 10-15 minutes.

Remove and de-bone the fresh fish. Add all other ingredients to the pot and bring sauce to a boil, stirring occasionally. Return the fish to the pot and simmer the sauce for another 10-15 minutes. This sauce can be eaten as a soup or poured over rice or millet couscous.[5]

Flower Salad

Moringa flowers
Seasonings
Oil
Vinegar

Steam the flowers, then add normal salad seasonings, oil and vinegar.[3]

"Pea Soup"

Moringa pods
Onion
Flour
Salt
Pepper

Slice open the older pods. Boil in water until soft. Then scrape out the seeds and white fleshy lining. Discard the rinds. The fleshy lining may be eaten as is (add spices for flavor) or returned to the water to help make the soup. Add onions, salt and pepper for flavor, add flour to thicken.[6]

Moringa Lentil Soup

Moringa pods
Lentils

A soup popular in India is made by slicing the older pods into 2" lengths and boiling in water along with lentils. Only the inside of the pod sections is eaten.[6]

Moringa Strips

Moringa pods
Seasonings to taste

Slice open the older pods and scrape out the fleshy lining, keeping the flesh intact (lightly boiling the pods beforehand will make this job easier). Strips of fleshy lining can be steamed and mixed with onions and spices. Strips can be fried in oil. Or strips can be added to other recipes.[6]

References

[1] Provided by Dr. Titia Warndorff in Binga, Zimbabwe.

[2] Provided by Salikou Ouattara of AMAPROS in Bamako, Mali.

[3] Provided by Martin Mané of AGADA in Ziguinchor, Senegal.

[4] Meitzner, L. and M. Price. Amaranthe to Zai Holes: Ideas for Growing Food Under Difficult Conditions. ECHO. North Fort Myers, Florida. pp 111-114. 1996

[5] Provided by Macodou Sow of APADEC in Tambacounda, Senegal.

[6] Provided by Martin Mané, also Meitzner and Price.

IF YOU'VE TRIED MORINGA, WHAT WAS YOUR EXPERIENCE?

Moringa is so new in America that few people have very much experience with it. What you read here is most of what is known about this remarkable tree.

We need a much broader base of real-world experience. I'm inviting you to share yours.

What kind of benefits did you notice? Any difficulties? A new recipe? Did you give Moringa to a friend or relative—what was their experience?

Share it with me. And let me know if I should keep it private—or if it's OK to include you in my next book or website update.

Send your experience to:
Sandy@LifeOnNet.org
Fax: 818-386-9102
14622 Ventura Blvd., #800
Sherman Oaks, CA 91403

Be in good health!

IF YOU HAVE A STORE
OR MARKET

Several wholesalers supply Moringa pods ("drumsticks") and other Moringa products to retailers. If you are aware of others, please let me know, but here are some to get you started.

India Imports and Exports Inc.
3838 West 102nd Street
Inglewood, CA 90303
Tel: (310) 330-8900

House of Spices
127-40 Willets Point Blvd.
Flushing, NY 11368
Tel: (718) 507-4600
Fax: (718) 507-4798

Sri Lankan Delight
19016 Ventura Blvd.
Tarzana, CA 91356
Tel: (818) 774-1237
Fax: (818) 774-1536

How to Plant, Grow and Harvest

*T*he first step in planting, growing and harvesting Moringa is to obtain some good seeds or a cutting from a healthy Moringa tree. Since cuttings are rarely used, let's look at seeds first.

Fortunately, these trees produce a large number of seeds. If you or a friend have a Moringa tree growing in a pot at home or out in the yard, let one of the pods grow to maturity. When a pod changes from green to brown and gets hard on the outside, it's probably ready. If the sides of the pod start to split open, it's definitely ready. As you crack open the pod, you should be rewarded with a handful of seeds, each of which can produce a new tree.

If you don't know someone with a Moringa tree, that's OK. I'll show you several places where you can order seeds.

Planting

Each seed should be planted about an inch deep in loosened soil. Often, this planting takes place indoors. One reason for this is

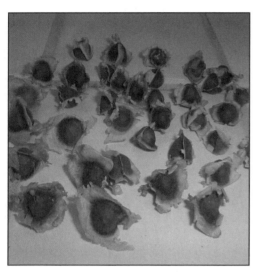

Moringa seeds

that while the germination rate is fairly high—about 80% for fresh seeds—the rate goes down to about 50% for seeds which have been stored for many months. Since not every seed germinates, it's best to plant in small containers first, then transplant them when you are sure you have a robust plant.

The second reason is the short growing season in those parts of the world where frosts occur. By starting the plant indoors, it will already have grown to a good height before the weather warms up and it's safe to move it outside.

The third reason for planting indoors is that many people have no yard, or live in an area where temperatures or soil conditions aren't suitable for growing the tree outside. If this is to be a permanent indoor plant, put it in the largest pot you can reasonably accommodate. This will give its roots the most room to grow.

You might ask, "How is it possible to grow a tree indoors?" Especially since, in its natural habitat, Moringa grows into a thin tree about 35 feet high. Even when it is grown outdoors, though, a tree that tall would be of little use, since the parts you want to harvest—the leaves, flowers and pods—would be far out of reach. As a result, people who cultivate Moringa trees—indoors or out— begin harvesting the top of the plant when it gets to be about 3 or 4 feet tall. This causes it to grow into a bushy plant where all of its natural gifts are within easy reach.

Since you're going to have a tree that's only 5 or 6 feet tall at the most, it can easily be grown indoors.

The basic requirements are soil, light and water.

Moringa grows best in soil that drains well. A sandy loam is best, but you can make other soils work. This is done by adding amendments such as peat moss, sand and compost. For indoors planting, I've found potting soil works very well. I use a mixture that includes aged and processed softwood bark and sawdust, sphagnum peat moss, perlite and pumice, composted animal manures, bat guano and kelp meal.

Moringa grows so fast that it quickly outgrows almost any pot. For that reason, I start by planting the seeds in pots made of Irish peat. When it comes time to move to a bigger pot or move the young tree outdoors, I just plant the entire peat pot in the soil. The peat eventually dissolves into the surrounding dirt, and the move to a new location is accomplished without ever disturbing the delicate roots.

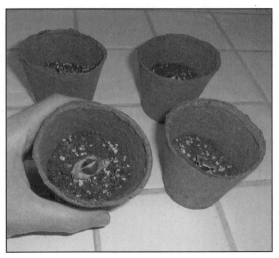

Whatever pot you use, begin by placing soil in the bottom of it to about 1¼ inches from the top. Lay one Moringa seed on top of the dirt, then cover it with another 1 inch of soil.

Water the soil daily until the young plant becomes visible.

Planting in peat pots

This will take about 2 weeks. Add only enough water to keep the soil moist, and avoid making puddles. Standing water can kill the tree.

That's another reason why I like using peat pots. Any excess water is absorbed by the pot and is easily visible as a dark area. Ideally, the outside of the peat pot should always be partially wet and partially dry. When the sprout is a few inches high, you can cut back to fewer waterings.

When the seed sprouts, place the pot near a bright window. The tree needs direct sunlight to grow well.

If your seeds are being planted out-doors, or if the small plant is being brought outside in the spring-time, pick a sunny spot where the tree will have room to grow.

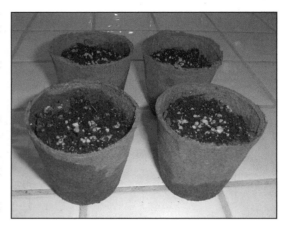

Seeds covered and watered

Since you'll be trimming the tree so it's only about 5 or 6 feet tall, you'll want to make sure there are no buildings or walls between it and the sunlight, and no taller, overhanging trees which will cast a shadow over the Moringa.

Equally important is the ground in which it's planted. Make sure the soil has been loosened by digging an area 2 feet wide and 2 to 3 feet deep. If necessary, amend the soil as described for indoor plants.

Watering is similar also, until the seed sprouts or the trans-plant takes root (about two weeks). At that point, the tree can survive on its own without additional watering. If you're in the middle of a very dry season though, occasional watering is fine.

Plant Growth

This is the fastest-growing tree I have ever seen. When left unharvested, it can grow 15 feet high in a single year.

After you see the small green plant poke its head out of the soil, it will only be a couple of months before it's 3 feet high. At this point, I recommend you clip the top of the tree. This will produce your first harvest. But equally as important, it will encourage the tree to branch out and produce more limbs. By the time your Moringa is 5 or 6 months old it will probably be about 5 feet tall, and that's as big as you want it to get.

Later, in addition to trimming the top of the tree, you'll want to shorten the tree limbs. This will cause the tree to make more limbs, and give it a bushy appearance. More limbs means more leaves, flowers and pods. A good rule of thumb for trimming tree limbs is: each time a limb grows another two feet long, cut it back one foot. You'll like the results.

After about 8 months the tree puts out its first flowers. After that it will continue to flower—off and on—year round.

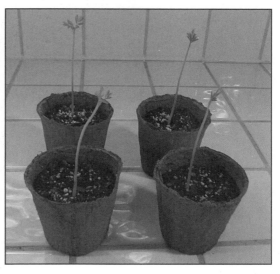

Plants germinate in about 2 weeks

At first you're likely to see only a few pods on the young tree. But as it establishes itself, the yield of leaves, flowers and pods goes up considerably. In India, a mature tree—which is cut back after each harvest so that it produces many branches—can yield 400 to 1000 pods per year.

While fertilizing the tree is not necessary, spreading steer manure around the base of the tree in early Spring seems to increase the yield. If you're raising the tree indoors, this is not recommended, or your family may place you and the tree outside.

As previously mentioned, outdoor trees don't usually need to be watered. This is because the main root tends to grow down to the water table and supply itself nicely. However, if conditions are dry and the growth of new leaves seems to be slowing down, watering the tree occasionally will keep it producing a bountiful harvest.

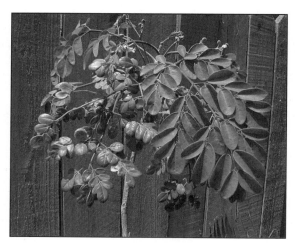

Moringa grows quickly

Actually, Moringa loves water. It needs at least 10 inches of rainfall a year, and does quite well up to 120 inches per year. The problem people sometimes encounter is that they don't have the loose, sandy loam which allows water to drain through quickly away from the roots. If you have heavy, clay-like soil, the water doesn't flow through the soil easily. If there's too much water, it tends to puddle around the roots. Moringa is amazingly resistant to insects and diseases. Its one weakness is root rot if left in standing water.

Since the appropriate amount of water varies with your particular soil conditions and humidity, I suggest you try a conservative amount of watering and watch to see how your tree grows. When you discover what works best in your environment, stick with it—and enjoy the results.

Temperature can also be significant. When Moringa grows outdoors, it's usually able to endure light frosts without harm. Freezes, however, may cause it to die back to ground level. Even then, new sprouts are likely to form from the roots, and the tree grows back quite rapidly.

Starting with Cuttings

As mentioned earlier, the other way to start growing Moringa, instead of using seeds, is to begin with a cutting taken from a mature tree. This requires a fairly substantial piece of the limb or trunk of the tree. The best cuttings are 1½ to 5 feet in length, and from 1½ to 6 inches in diameter. It is recommended that the cutting be left to dry in a shady place for three days before planting.

The cutting can be planted indoors or outside, with the same temperature, soil and water conditions that apply to seeds.

To plant the cutting, make sure the soil has been loosened by digging an area 2 feet wide and 2 to 3 feet deep. Amend the soil as described earlier. Plant one third of the length of the cutting under ground (the thicker end).

Water the cutting daily until you start to see green growth beginning to bud from the cutting. After that, watering for outdoor trees is optional, depending on how wet or dry your climate conditions are. Indoors, watering the cutting every second or third day should be sufficient after it takes root. In each case, only add enough water to allow moisture to reach the roots but not to form puddles around them.

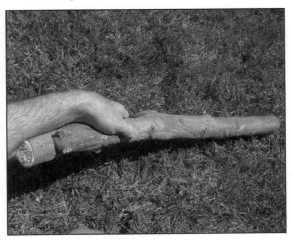

Cuttings are usually over 1½ inches thick

It is generally believed that cuttings will result in faster growth than planting from seeds, but the roots tend to be more shallow and therefore less drought-tolerant. There is open debate as to whether these trees produce superior or inferior pods compared to trees grown from seeds. Since no one can prove their point, there's probably no significant difference in the pods produced.

When grown from a cutting, you can expect the new tree to begin bearing pods about 6 to 8 months after it was planted.

Harvesting

Moringa is a bountiful tree. It produces three yields instead of just one. You get to harvest the leaves, as well as the pods and flowers. There is always something on the tree for you, all year long.

Leaves

Most plentiful are the leaves, which are always green, tender and ready to eat. They are best when eaten fresh, so just before mealtime you can walk over to the tree and take what you need. The tree grows so quickly that it readily replaces whatever you use.

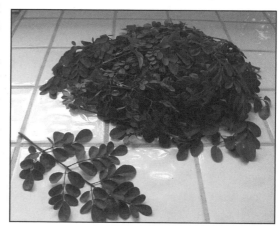

Harvested leaves

Normally, the only time other than meal-time when you harvest leaves is when you're cutting the tree back to keep it from getting too tall or shortening some of the tree limbs to cause more branches to form. At tree-trimming time you usually end up with a huge pile of leaves, more than you could ever hope to eat while they're still fresh. This is the ideal time to make leaf powder.

One of the great things about leaf powder is that you can store it for long periods of time and use it whenever you want. So making a big harvest and producing a stockpile of powder is a great idea.

Also, for your friends who would like to get the benefit of Moringa but don't have their own tree, you can make small gift-packets of leaf powder. As the tree gets larger, your harvests will be huge, so you can afford it. And the gifts are treasured!

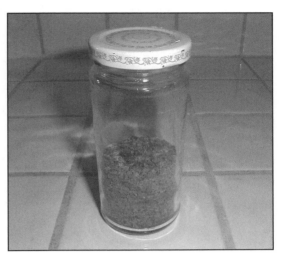

Leaf powder

Pods

The pods are harvested at four different times.

When they are small, green and tender, they're perfect for any recipe in which you would use green beans. And they have their own nutritional benefit which is different than the leaves. As before, these are best when picked fresh just before the meal.

As the pods get larger and the outside

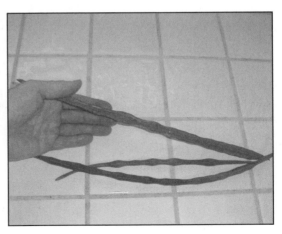

Harvested pods

covering gets harder, you move into the next harvest window. Pods taken at this time are used for the edible seeds inside. At this stage the seeds are quite tender and can be included in recipes just as you would use peas. For this use also, it's best to pick the pods just before mealtime, to experience them at their freshest and tastiest.

The third harvest opportunity is when the pods are fully mature. At this point, the outside casing has gotten brown and quite hard. What you're gathering now are seeds which can be used for planting and growing new Moringa trees. As you crack open the pod you'll see dark brown seeds inside. They should be stored in a dry, shady place until you're ready to use them.

The final pod harvest coincides with tree-trimming. Just like with the leaves, this harvest is usually much more than you can reasonably use while it's still fresh. This is a great time to think of your friends and neighbors. Moringa is so new, it's still very hard to find these health-enhancing pods. Due to the tree-trimming, you're like likely to have plenty of tender green pods, harder pods and a fresh supply of mature seeds ready for planting. It's a great time to share!

Flowers

Flowers are abundant on the Moringa tree. As nearly as I can tell, the tree uses whichever flower first begins to produce a pod, and sheds all the others on that part of the limb. So you might as well pick all the flowers you want. Just be careful to avoid the tiny pods you see developing.

While the flowers are supposed to have only two growing seasons a year, that seems to cover a fairly substantial part of

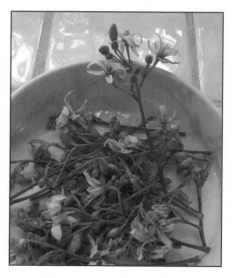

Harvested flowers

the year, so you're frequently able to find flowers when you want them.

I mostly use the flowers to make a nice, relaxing tea. This seems to be best when the flowers are fairly fresh. Some people apparently use dried flowers, which means they can harvest them in season and use them all year. You can go with whatever works best for you.

Where to Buy Seeds

As mentioned earlier, the best way to get started with Moringa is to get seeds or a cutting from a friend. That also strengthens the bond between you because people always remember where they got this remarkable gift. It also gives you a good source of practical information on raising and using your healthy harvest.

However, Moringa is still so new in the developed world that you'll be hard pressed to find it in your neighborhood. In fact, you'd probably be a leader in this adventure by raising one of the first Moringa trees in the area, then sharing its bounty with envious neighbors and friends who find out about the nutritional goldmine you have.

You could try calling tree nurseries, but so far I've yet to find anyone who sells the trees already grown. Eventually they will, of course, once they realize people are discovering it.

All of this means you probably need a good source of Moringa seeds. Fortunately, I've found quite a few. I can't guarantee the quality of the seeds everyone sends out, but Moringa seeds are pretty hardy and grow easily, so you shouldn't have any trouble.

USA – ECHO

One of the best sources for Moringa seeds is the Educational Concerns for Hunger Organization (ECHO). Their caring programs and dedicated efforts are described in other chapters.

You can read about the seeds on their web page, then get the order form on-line. At this point you still have to mail or fax the form to them. You'll find the people at ECHO to be very familiar with Moringa, and exceptionally helpful. They keep a large supply of Moringa seeds and respond very promptly.

ECHO
17391 Durrance Road
N. Fort Myers, FL 33917
Tel: 941-543-3246
Fax: 941-543-5317
Email: echo@echonet.org
Web: www.echonet.org/usseed.htm

USA – Seedman

Jim Johnson's company, Seedman, provides seeds from around the world. Orders can be placed by mail, fax, email or Internet. Their recent price was $1.95 per pack of 5 Moringa seeds, but they were out at the time I talked with them. Very nice people, they only accept orders when they have seeds in stock. They can be reached at:

Seedman
3421 Bream Street
Gautier, MS 39553
Tel: 800-336-2064
Fax: 228-497-5488
Email: seedman@seedman.com
Web: http://seedman.com

USA – Peace Seeds

This small but ecologically conscious group can also supply you with seeds. Contact:

Peace Seeds
2385 S.E. Thompson Street
Corvallis, OR 97333
Tel: 541-753-7333
Fax: 541-753-0604

International Calls

All telephone numbers shown are for calls from the United States. If you're calling to the USA from another country, add 01 to the front of the number. If you are in the country (other than the USA) listed here, drop the 011 and 2-or-3 digit country code and dial a 0 first, then the number as shown.

Kenya

Dr. David Odee
Head Biotechnology Division
Kenya Forestry Research Institute
P.O. Box 20412
Nairobi, Kenya
Tel: 011 254 154-32891
Fax: 011 254 154-32844
Email: kefri@arcc.or.ke   Put "Attn David Odee"
                                 on the subject line.

New Zealand

Peter B. Dow & Co.
P.O. Box 696
Grisborne 3800
New Zealand
Fax: 011 64 79-78844

Australia

Ellison Horticultural PTY, Ltd.
P.O. Box 365
Nowra, N.S.W. 2541
Australia
Tel: 011 61 44-214255

India

Kumar International
Ajitmal 206121
Etawah, Uttar Pradesh
India

Singapore

Samuel Ratnam
Inland & Foreign Trading Co.
Block 79A, Indus Road #04-418/420
Singapore
Tel: 011 65 316-272-2711
Fax: 011 65 316-271-6118

Botanical Information

Division: Magnoliophyta

Class: Magnoliopsida

Subclass: Dilleniidae

Order: Capparidales

Family: Moringaceae

Species: *Moringa oleifera*

Moringa oleifera is the best known and most nutritionally valuable species of Moringa. That is what I raise, and those are the seeds you're most likely to find.

The other members of the Moringa family are divided into three groups by Mark Olson, who has done extensive research on Moringa.[1] Those groups are: slender trees; bottle trees; and the shrubs, herbs and trees of Northeast Africa. In each case, "M." is the abbreviation for Moringa. The countries in which it is currently found in nature are also noted.

Slender Trees

These are thin trees with a tuberous juvenile stage and cream to pink, slightly bilaterally-symmetrical flowers.

M. oleifera – India

M. concanensis – India, Pakistan, Bangladesh

M. peregrina – Red Sea, Arabia, Horn of Africa

Bottle Trees

These are massive trees with bloated, water-storing trunks and small radially symmetrical flowers.

M. drouhardii – Madagascar

M. hildebrandtii – Madagascar

M. ovalifolia – Namibia and SW Angola

M. stenopetala – Kenya and Ethiopia

Shrubs, Herbs and Trees of NE Africa

These are tuberous adults or tuberous juveniles maturing to fleshy-rooted adults and have colorful, bilaterally symmetrical flowers.

M. arborea – NE Kenya

M. borziana – Kenya and Somalia

M. longituba – Ethiopia, Kenya, Somalia

M. pygmaea – N Somalia

M. rivae – Kenya and Ethiopia

M. ruspoliana – Ethiopia, Kenya, Somalia

Apparently M. oleifera is sometimes, though incorrectly, referred to as *M. aptera* and *M. pterygosperma*.

Description

Moringa oleifera, the most popular member of this family, is a slender, deciduous tree which grows to about 30 feet in height. It develops a large base with age, and has tuberous roots. The stem and branches are brittle, with corky bark.

The leaves are feathery, green and fern-like in appearance. They are pinnately compound, which means they have small, oval-shaped leaflets on each side of the stem.

The flower buds are pink on the outside, opening to reveal white or creamy white petals and yellow stamens.

The pods are pendulous, triangular in cross-section, green when young, which grow brown as they age. They typically grow to about 12 - 16 inches long (though some varieties are as long as 4 feet), and ¾ to 1¼ inches in diameter, tapering at both ends. They are called "kachang kelur" in Singapore and "drumsticks" in English. The pods split lengthwise into 3 parts when dry, revealing seeds embedded in the pith. The mature seeds are dark brown, with 3 papery wings.

The pungent scent in all parts of the plant is distinctive.

Moringa was originally thought to be suitable only for altitudes from sea level to 2000 feet, and probably flourishes best in that range. However varieties have been discovered at altitudes of 4000 feet in Mexico and above 6500 feet in Zimbabwe.

It has adapted to a wide range of soil types, but does best in a well-drained, sandy loam. Heavier clay soils will be tolerated, as long as water-logging is avoided. Moringa prefers a neutral to slightly acidic soil, but it has been grown successfully on Pacific atolls where soil pH is often greater than 8.5.

It does best where temperatures range from 70° to 100°F, but will tolerate even a light frost. A freeze typically kills the tree to the ground, though it will grow back from the roots. Moringa prefers annual rainfalls over 20 inches, but will grow with at least 10 inches. It has been known to tolerate up to 120 inches of rain annually.

Nutritional Value

The following analysis of Moringa pods, fresh leaves and dried leaf powder was provided by Fuglie.[2] He in turn had obtained the information on pods and fresh leaves from Booth and Wickens.[3] The analysis of leaf powder was sponsored by CWS and the Department of Engineering at the University of Leicester, and was performed by Campden & Chorleywood Food Research Association. Some of the differences between the fresh and dried leaf content were due to the fact that the leaves which were tested came from different sources.

Nutritional Value Chart

Per 100 grams of edible portion:	Pods	Leaves	Leaf Powder
Water (%)	86.9	75.0	7.5
Calories	26	92	205
Protein (g)	2.5	6.7	27.1
Fat (g)	0.1	1.7	2.3
Carbohydrate (g)	3.7	13.4	38.2
Fiber (g)	4.8	0.9	19.2
Minerals (g)	2.0	2.3	-
Ca (mg)	30	440	2003
Mg (mg	24	24	368
P (mg)	110	70	204
K (mg)	259	259	1324
Cu (mg)	3.1	1.1	0.57
Fe (mg)	5.3	7.0	28.2
S (g)	137	137	870
Oxalic acid (mg)	10	101	1.6
Vitamin A – Beta carotene (mg)	0.11	6.8	16.3
Vitamin B – choline (mg)	423	423	-
Vitamin B_1 – thiamin (mg)	0.05	0.21	2.64
Vitamin B_2 – riboflavin (mg)	0.07	0.05	20.5
Vitamin B_3 – nicotinic acid (mg)	0.2	0.8	8.2
Vitamin C – ascorbic acid (mg)	120	220	17.3
Vitamin E – tocopherol acetate	-	-	113
Arginine (g/16g N)	3.6	6.0	1.33%
Histidine (g/16g N)	1.1	2.1	0.61%
Lysine (g/16g N)	1.5	4.3	1.32%
Tryptophan (g/16g N)	0.8	1.9	0.43%
Phenylanaline (g/16g N)	4.3	6.4	1.39%
Methionine (g/16g N)	1.4	2.0	0.35%
Threonine (g/16g N)	3.9	4.9	1.19%
Leucine (g/16g N)	6.5	9.3	1.95%
Isoleucine (g/16g N)	4.4	6.3	0.83%
Valine (g/16g N)	5.4	7.1	1.06%

The following analysis of Moringa seed kernels was provided by James A. Duke.[4] He noted that the kernel makes up 70-74% of the seed.

Per 100 g, the seed kernel contains 4.08 water, 38.4 g crude protein, 34.7% fatty oil, 16.4 g N free extract, 3.5 g fiber, and 3.2 g ash. The seed oil contains fatty acids as described in the following section. The cake left after oil extraction contains 58.9% crude protein, 0.4 % CaO, 1.1 % P_2O_5 and 0.8% K_2O.

Seed Oil

According to John Sutherland at the University of Leicester in England,[5] interest in the oil extracted from *Moringa oleifera*, known commercially as Ben oil, has existed for almost 200 years. In 1817 a petition containing particulars relating to the oil from M. oleifera was presented to the Jamaican House of Assembly. The petition described the oil as being useful for salads and culinary purposes and to be equal to the best Florence oil as an illuminant giving a clear light without smoke.

A subsequent paper presented to the Jamaica Society of Arts in 1854 described how samples of oil had been tested by two watch-making establishments in Kingston and had been reported to be equal to the expensively imported "watch oil." Subsequent reports indicated that the oil was used extensively as a lubricant until being replaced by sperm-whale oil.

The oil has also been reported to have been used extensively in the "enfleurage" process whereby delicate fragrances are extracted from flower petals.

The first recorded study of the composition of the oil was carried out in 1848 which revealed a fatty acid with a high melting point. This was subsequently called behenic acid, from which the commercial name for M. oleifera oil came.

The oil produced is pale yellow in color, non-drying with a mild, characteristic nutty flavor. The seed kernel contains on average 40% oil by weight. The composition of the oil is considered to be similar to that for olive oil and as such is considered suitable for similar purposes.

An analysis of M. oleifera oil by NRI in 1993 revealed the following distribution of fatty acids: 72.9% oleic, 7.3% behenic, 5.9% palmitic, 5.1% stearic, 3.6% arachidic, 2.3% eicosenoic, 1.1% palitoleic, 1.0% lignoceric, 0.6% linoleic, 0.1%linolenic, 0.1% myristic.

Popular Local Names

Moringa is the universal name for this tree, but it is also known by other names in different languages, including:

English	Drumstick tree	
	Horseradish tree	
French	Ben aile	
	Benzolive	
India	Sajna	(Bengali)
	Suragavo	(Gujarati)
	Shajmah, Shajna, Segra	(Hindi)
	Sigru, Moringa, Muringa	(Malayam)
	Sujna, Shevga	(Marathi)
	Munigha, Sajina	(Oriya)
	Sanjina, Soanjana	(Punjabese)
	Sobhan Jana	(Sanskrit)
	Murungai, Murunkak-kai	(Tamil)
	Sajana	(Telegu)
Burma	Dandalonbin	
Cambodia	Daem mrum	
Indonesia	Kalor, Kelor	

Philippines	Malunkai, Malunggay	
	Mulangai, Mulangay	
Sri Lanka	Murunga	
Kenya	Mlonge, Mronge, Mrongo	(Swahili)
	Mlongo, Mzunze, Mzungu	"
Malawi	Cham'mwanba, Kangaluni	(Chichewa)
	Kalokola	(Yao)
	Nsangoa	(Senna)
Niger	Zogala gandi	(Hausa)
	Windi-bundu	(Zarma)
Burkina Faso	Argentiga, Arzam tigha	(More)
	Guilgandani, Gigandjah	(Fulfulde)
Ghana	Yevu-ti	(Ewe)
Nigeria	Gawara, Konamarade	(Fulani)
	Rini maka, Habiwal hausa	"
	Zogall, Zogalla-gandi	(Hausa)
	Bagaruwar-maka, -masar	"
	Shipka hali, Shuka halinka	"
	Barambo, Koraukin zaila	"
	Rimin-turawa, -nacara	"
	Ikwe oyibo	(Ibo)
	Ewe ile, Ewe igbale	(Yoruba)
	Idagbo monoye	"
Senegal	Neverday	(Wolof)
	Nebeday	(Serer)
Sudan	Ruwag, Alim, Halim	(Arabic)
	Shagara al-ruwag, -rauwaq	"
Togo	Baganlua, bagaelean	(Dagomba)
Zimbabwe	Mupulanga, Zakalanda	(Tonga)
Colombia	Angela	

Costa Rico	Marango
Cuba	Palo Jeringa, Palo de Tambor
Dominican Rep.	Palo de aceiti, Palo de abejas
	Libertad
El Salvador	Teberinto
Guadalupe	Moloko
Guatamala	Perlas, Paraiso blanco
Guiana	Saijhan
Haiti	Benzolive, Benzolivier
	Ben oleifere, Graines benne
	Bambou-bananier
Honduras	Maranga calalu
Panama	Jacinto
Puerto Rico	Resada, Ben, Jasmin frances
Surinam	Peperwortel boom
Other	Acacia, Aceite, Aljian-tija
	Alsan-tiiga, Arbol de las perlas
	Arbol do los asparagos, Arzantija
	Bamboubamamoer, Benaile
	Benbom, Benboom, Brenoili
	Cedro, Cenauro, Chinto borrego
	Chuva de prata, Desengano
	Gailito, Goma, Guairena
	Guilgandeni, Hoja de sen
	Kpatovigb, Legi-lakili
	Macasar, Maloko, Marenque
	Moongay, Moriengo, Naragno
	Noz de bem, Orenga, Orselli
	Palo de geringa, Palo jeringa
	Paraiso, Paraiso de espana

Paraiso extranjero, Paraiso frances
Perlas del oriente, Pois quinique
Quiabo de tres quinas, Sainto John
Salaster, Salibau, Sen, Seringa
Yevovigb.

References

[1] http://hoya.mobot.org/gradstudents/olson/moringahome.html

[2] Fuglie, L.J. The Miracle Tree: *Moringa oleifera*, Natural Nutrition for the Tropics. Church World Service. Dakar, Senegal. 1999

[3] Booth, F.E.M. and G.E. Wickens. "Non-timber uses of selected arid zone trees and shrubs in Africa". FAO Conservation Guide. pp 92-101. Rome. 1988

[4] Duke, J.A. Handbook of Energy Corps (unpublished). 1983

[5] www.le.ac.uk/engineeering/staff/Sutherland/moringa/moringa.htm

Research & Websites
Around the World

*T*o help create a clearinghouse of information available on Moringa, I've been gathering research papers, websites, articles and books from all over the world. Most of them are listed here and in the Bibliography for your use. If you have any additional sources and are willing to share them with other health-conscious people, please email them to me at Sandy@LifeOnNet.org.

You can find new updates
posted at this website:

www.LifeOnNet.org/moringa.html

An excellent example of good research belongs to Mark Olson. Mark did his PhD dissertation on Moringa at Washington University and collected an extensive amount of information on the different species of the Moringa family. He posted those findings—with photographs—on his website:

http://hoya.mobot.org/gradstudents/olson/moringahome.html

I mentioned to him the many varieties of Moringa being bred by growers in India to meet special needs such as higher yields, different-sized pods and shorter tree height, and wondered if any of these could be considered a new species.

He indicated that these are "breeds" of Moringa, in the same way that there are breeds of dogs, but all stay in their original species. In the plant world, instead of breeds, these are called "cultivars," which is short for cultivated varieties.

Mark can be reached at olsonm@mobot.mobot.org

At the University of Leicester in England, Dr. Geoff Folkard and John Sutherland and have done excellent work with Moringa for many years, producing a series of papers.

Dr. Folkard is a recognized authority on the use of Moringa for water purification. He has written about Moringa being used for this purpose by individuals, and also about facilities which service an entire village.

I asked which method he thought would be pursued as having the most benefit, and he said both have about the same potential at this point. In support of that, he mentioned an excellent "home" water treatment project in Brazil using Moringa...and also that there is a company trying to extract the active coagulant proteins from Moringa for commercial use.

He can be reached at:

Dr. Geoff Folkard
Department of Engineering
University of Leicester
University Road
Leicester LE1 7RH
UK
Tel: 011 44 116-252-2538

Fax: 011 44 116-252-2619
Email: gkf@le.ac.uk

John Sutherland, also at the University of Leicester, presents some of his and Dr. Folkard's work, plus references to other sources, on a very thorough collection of web pages which you can access at:

www.le.ac.uk/engineering/staff/Sutherland/moringa/moringa.htm

He can be reached at the above address and at:
Tel: 011 44 116-252-5271
Fax: 011 44 116-252-2619
Email: spj@leicester.ac.uk

Dr. Samia Al Azharia Jahn with the Deutsche Gesellschaft fur Technische Zusammenarbeit (GTZ) in Germany has produced a number of excellent technical bulletins on Moringa. She can be contacted at:

Dr. S.A.A. Jahn
GTZ, FB 332
Dag-Hammarskjold-Weg 1-2
Postfach 5180
D-6236 Eschborn 1 bei Frankfort/Main
Germany

Lowell J. Fuglie's work in Senegal, has already been described in several earlier chapters. I asked him recently if he thought his project to introduce Moringa in areas of serious health needs and malnutrition could be successfully implemented in other areas as well.

He told me it probably could, but would need to be modified to fit the culture of each country. It would be easiest in countries where it is already part of the local diet to some degree. In other countries he thought using the leaf powder as an additive might be the easiest way to introduce it.

He added, "Even in countries where Moringa is not eaten, it is often widely used in traditional medicines so people have a certain esteem for the tree's qualities."

He can be reached at:

Lowell J. Fuglie
Church World Service
12 rue Felix Faure
B.P. 3822
Dakar, Senegal
Tel: 011 221 822-43-40
Fax: 011 221 821-63-84
Email: fuglie@sonatel.senet.net

See the chapter on Helping the World's Needy for information on the services, research, address, telephone, fax, email and website information for these three organizations:

⊠   ECHO

⊠   Trees for Life

⊠   NCC/CWS

Purdue University provides a good jumping-off point to find two excellent on-line documents: the Handbook of Energy Crops by James A. Duke, and New Crops: Solutions for Global Problems by Noel Vietmeyer. You start at:

http://newcrop.hort.purdue.edu/newcrop/nexus/Moringa_oleifera_nex.html

University of Hawaii has information on Moringa at its website:

http://agrss.sherman.hawaii.edu/onfarm/tree/tree0012.html

At the University of New Orleans site, L. Watson and M.J. Dallwitz provide highly technical botanical information on Moringa. So far as I know, their extensive reference exists only on the Internet. You can see it at:

http://biodiversity.uno.edu/delta/angio/www/moringac.htm

University of Connecticut's Ecology & Evolutionary Biology Conservatory works with Moringa, and provides information on the Internet at:

http://florawww.eeb.uconn.edu/acc_num/199700027.html

Clinton Morse is the greenhouse manager at U. Conn's EEBC, and can be reached at:

Ecology &Evolutionary Biology Conservatory
75 North Eagleville Road
Box U-3043
Storrs, CA 06269
Tel: 860-486-0809   Office
Tel: 860-486-4052   Greenhouse
Fax: 860-486-6364

Ben Bazeley works on Moringa with Dr. Folkard in the United Kingdom, and can be contacted at:

Ben W. Bazeley
Stoneleigh
37 Sutton Road, Shrewsbury
Shropshire SY2 6DL

UK
Tel: 011 44 743-236-762

Dr Titia Warndorff performs awareness education about Moringa in Zimbabwe:

Dr. Titia Warndorff
Binga Trees Trust
Private Bag 5715
Binga, Zimbabwe
Tel: 011 263 15-321
Email: gwwarndorff@healthnet.zw

Susan van't Riet educates people in Malawi about the benefits of Moringa, and can be reached at:

Susan van't Riet
International Eye Foundation
P.O. Box 2273
Blantyre, Malawi
Email: ief@malawi.net

See the Bibliography for an extensive list of published information on Moringa from countries around the world.

Definitions

Alkaloid – *n.* organic, nitrogen-containing ring compound of vegetable origin which has a bitter taste. [1825-35; < AL-KAL(I) + OID < ME alkaly < MF alkali < dial. Ar al-qali]

Analgesic – *n.* a remedy that relieves pain. [1870-75; < ANAL-GES(IA) + IC < NL < Gk analgesia, painlessness]

Anthelmintic – *adj.* capable of eliminating parasitic worms. [1675-85; ANT + HELMINT(H)IC < Gk helminth, a kind of worm]

Antibiotic – *n.* chemical substance having the ability to inhibit or destroy bacteria and other microorganisms. [1855-60; ANTI + BIOTIC < Gk biotikos, pertaining to life]

Antipyretic – *adj.* checking or preventing fever. [1675-85; ANTI + PYRETIC < NL pyreticus, pertaining to fever]

Aqueous – *adj.* containing water, watery. [1635-45; AQU(A) + EOUS < L: water]

Articular – *adj.* pertaining to the joints. [1400-50; late ME < L ARTICULAR(IS)]

Calculous – *adj.* characterized by the presence of stone. [1400-50; late ME calculose, full of stones < L CALCUL(OSUS) + OUS having small stones]

Caries – *n.* decay. [1625-35; < L CARIES decay]

Carminative – *n.* a drug causing expulsion of gas from the stomach or bowel. [1645-55; < LL CARMINAT(US) + IVE purified]

Catarrh – *n.* inflammation of a mucous membrane accompanied by excessive secretions. [1350-1400; ME < LL CATARRH(US) < Gk katarrous, down-flowing]

Diuretic – n. a medicine which increases urine flow. [1375-1425; ME d(i)uretik < LL DIURETIC(US) < Gk diouretikos, urinate]

Extract – *n.* a substance drawn out from a plant or other source which contains its essence. [1375-1425; late ME < L EXTRACT(US)]

Hypoglycemic – *adj.* pertaining to an abnormally low amount of glucose in the blood. [1890-95; HYPO + GLYC + EMIA]

Infusion – *n.* the liquid prepared by soaking a leaf, bark or other substance in water. [1400-50; late ME < L INFUSION, a pouring into]

Inhibition – *n.* the act of restraining. [1350-1400; ME inhibicio(u)n < L INHIBITION held]

In vitro – performed in a laboratory vessel rather than in a living organism. [1890-95; < L IN VITRO in glass]

Lectin – *n.* a group of proteins that bind to particular carbohydrates in the manner of an antibody. [1954; < L LECT(US) + IN gather]

Malnutrition – *n.* lack of food or nutriment needed for proper health or growth. [1860-65; MAL + NUTRITION]

Pedal edema – *n.* accumulation of serious fluid in the tissues of the foot. [1605-15; < L PEDAL(IS) (O)EDEMA swelling of the foot]

Poultice – *n.* a moist mass of herbs or other substance applied hot as a medication to the body. [1535-45; < pultes < L puls]

Purgative – *n.* a medicine or agent which removes whatever is impure or undesirable. [1350-1400; < LL PURGATIV(US) + E making clean]

Rubefacient – *n.* a medicinal application which causes a redness of the skin. [1795-1805; < L RUBEFACIENT reddening]

Stimulant – *n.* something which temporarily quickens some vital process. [1720-30; < L STIMULANT goaded]

Tonic – *n.* a medicine that invigorates or strengthens. [1640-50; < Gk TONI(KOS) + C, pertaining to stretching]

Trauma – *n.* shock or wound produced by sudden physical injury. [1685-95; < Gk TRAUMA wound]

Vagus nerve – *n.* either one of the tenth pair of cranial nerves. [1830-40]

Vesicant – *n.* a substance which produces a blister. [1655-65; < NL VESICANT]

Bibliography

Agbessi Dos-Santos, H. and M. Damon. (In French) Manuel de Nutrition Africaine. Institut Panafricain pour le Developpement. Douala, Cameroun. 1987

Anon. "The nature and commercial uses of Ben oil". Supplement to the Board of Trade Journal, Bulletin of the Imperial Institute. pp 117-120. 1904

Baker, H.M. Nutrition and Dietetics for Health Care. Ninth Edition. Churchill Livingstone. New York. 1996

Bazeley, B.W. "The Moringa: a miracle tree for developing countries?" The Rotarian. February, pp. 6-7. 1999

Besse, F. (In French) *"Moringa oleifera*: L'arbre du mois". Le Flamboyant. Reseau Arbres Tropicaux, Silva. Nogent-sur-Marne, France. December, 40. 1996

Booth, F.E.M. and G.E. Wickens "Non-timber uses of selected arid zone trees and shrubs in Africa". FAO Conservation Guide. pp 92-101. Rome. 1988

Briend, A. (In French) Prevention et Traitment de la Malnutrition. Orstom. Dakar, Senegal. 1985

Burkill, J.H. A Dictionary of Economic Products of the Maylay Peninsula. Art Printing Works. Kuala Lumpur. 1966

Busson, F. (In French) Plantes alimentaires de l'Ouest Africain. Leconte. Marseille, France. 1965

Caceres, A. "Pharmacological properties of *Moringa oleifera*. 3: Effect of seed extracts in the treatment of experimental pydermia". Fitoterapia. LXII(5), pp. 449-450. 1991

Caceres, A., O. Cabrera, O. Morales, P. Mollinedo and P. Mendia. "Pharmacological properties of *Moringa oleifera*. 1: Preliminary screening for antimicrobial activity". Journal of Ethnopharmacology. 33, pp. 213-216. 1990

Caceres, A., A. Saravia, S. Rizzo, Z. Lorena, E. DeLeon and F. Nave. "Pharmacologic properties of *Moringa oleifera*. 2: Screening for antispasmodic, anti-inflammatory and diuretic activity". Journal of Ethnopharmacology. 36: pp. 233-237. 1992

Campden & Chorleywood Food Research Association. Analysis of Leaf Powder for Nutritional Composition. Report on Findings. July 17, 1998

Dahot, M.U. and A.R. Memnon. "Nutritive significance of oil extracted from *Moringa oleifera* seeds". Journal of Pharmacy, University of Karachi. 3(2), pp 75-79. 1985

Dietz, M., R. Metzler and C. Zarate. "Food security in the village: the case of oilseed processing". Appropriate Technology. 20(4), pp 9-11. 1994

D'souza, J. and A.R. Kulkarni. "Comparative studies on nutritive values of tender foliage of seedlings and mature plants of *Moringa oleifera* Lam." Journal of Econ. Tax. Bot. 17(2), pp 479-485. 1993

Duke, J.A. Handbook of Energy Corps. (Unpublished document). 1983

Eilert, U., B. Wolters and A. Nahrstedt "The antibiotic principle of seeds of *Moringa oleifera* and *Moringa stenopetala*". Journal of Medicinal Plant Research. 42, pp 55-61. 1981

Ezeamuzie, I.C., A.W. Ambadederomo, F.O. Shode and S.C. Ekwebelem. "Anti-inflammatory effects of *Moringa oleifera* root extract". International Journal of Pharmacognosy. 34(3), pp. 207-212. 1996

Faizi, S., B.S. Siddiqui, R. Saleem, S. Siddiqui and K. Aftab "Isolation and structure elucidation of new nitrile and mustard oil glycosides from *Moringa oleifera* and their effect on blood pressure". Journal of Natural Products. 57(9), pp 1256-1261. 1994

Ferrao, A.M.B. and J.E.M. Ferrao. (In Spanish) "Acidos gordos em oleo de moringuerio". Agronomia Angolana. 30, pp 3-16. Luanda, Angola. 1970

Folkard, G.K. and J.P. Sutherland. "*Moringa oleifera*: a tree and a litany of potential". Agroforestry Today. 8(3) pp. 5-8. 1996

Folkard, G.K. and J.P. Sutherland. "*Moringa oleifera*: a multipurpose tree. Food Chain No. 18, July 1996". Intermediate Technology. Myson House, Railway Terrace, Rugby, UK 1996

Folkard, G.K., J.P. Sutherland and W.D. Grant. "Natural coagulants at pilot scale". In: J. Pickford ed. Water, Environment and Management: Proceedings of the 18th WEDC Conference, Kathmandu, Nepal, August 30-September 3, 1992. Loughborough University Press. pp 51-54. 1993

Folkard, G.K. and J.P. Sutherland. "Sustainability of Water and Sanitation Systems". Paper presented to the 21st WEDC Conference in Kampala, Uganda. 1995

Fuglie, L.J. The Miracle Tree: *Moringa oleifera*, Natural Nutrition for the Tropics. Church World Service. Dakar, Senegal. 1999

Fritz, M. "A common tree with rare power". Los Angeles Times. Page A1. March 27, 2000

Gassenschmidt, U., K.D. Jany, B. Tauscher and H. Niebergall. "Isolation and characterization of a flocculating protein from *Moringa oleifera* Lam." Biochimica et Biophysica Acta. 1243, pp 477-481. 1995

Gopalan et al. Nutritive Value of Indian Foods. National Institute of Nutrition, Indian Council of Medical Research. Hyderabad, India. 1971

Hartwell, J.L. "Plants used against cancer. A survey". Lloydia pp 30-34. 1967

Holmes, R.G.H., V.E. Travis, J.P. Sutherland and G.K. Folkard. "The use of natural coagulants to treat wastewater for agricultural re-use in developing countries". Paper presented at International Conference "Science and Technology in Third World Development", University of Strathclyde in April 1993. pp 39-47. Glasgow. 1993

Jahn, S.A.A. Traditional water purification in tropical developing countries: existing methods and potential applications. Manual No. 117. Pub: GTZ, Eschborn, Germany. 1981

Jahn, S.A.A. "*Moringa oleifera* for food and water purification—selection of clones and growing of annual short stem". Entwicklung & Landlicher Raum. 23(4), pp 22-25. 1989

Jamieson, G.S. "Ben (Moringa) seed oil". Oil and Soap. 16, pp 173-174. 1939

Jayavardhanan, K.K., K. Suresh, K.R. Panikkar and D.M. Vasudevan. "Modular potency of drumstick lectin on the host defense system". Journal of Experimental Clinical Cancer Research. 13(3), pp 205-209. 1994

Le Poole, H.A.C. "Behen oil: A classic oil for modern cosmetics". Cosmetics & Toiletries. p. 77. January 1996

Limaye D.A., A.Y. Nimbkar, R. Jain and M. Ahmad. "Cardiovascular effects of the aqueous extract of *Moringa pterygosperma*". Phytotherapy Research. 9, pp. 37-40. 1995

Madsen, M., J. Schlundt and O. El Fadil. "Effect of water coagulation by seeds of *Moringa oleifera* on bacterial concentrations". Journal of Tropical Medicine and Hygiene. 90: pp 101-109. 1987

Makonnen, E., A. Hunde and G. Damecha. "Hypoglycaemic effect of *Moringa stenopetala* aqueous extract in rabbits". Phytotherapy Research. 11, pp. 147-148. 1997

Martin, F.W. CRC Handbook of Tropical Food. CRC Press. 1984

McDonald, H.J. and F.M. Sapone. Nutrition for the Prime of Life: The Adult's Guide to Healthier Living. Insight Books, Plenem Press. New York. 1993

Meitzner, L. and M. Price. Amaranthe to Zai Holes: Ideas for Growing Food Under Difficult Conditions. ECHO. North Fort Myers, Florida. 1996

Mervyn, L. Thorson's Complete Guide to Vitamins & Minerals. Thorson's Publishing Ltd. UK. 1989

Morton, J.F. "The horseradish tree, *Moringa pterygosperma* (Moringaceae) – A boon to arid lands?" Economic Botany. 45(3), pp 318-333. 1991

Nath, P. "Drumstick Dossier". Swagat, Indian Airlines inflight magazine. January, p. 93. 1999

Nautiyal, B.P. and K.G. Venkataraman. "Moringa (drumstick) – an ideal tree for social forestry: growing conditions and uses – part 1". Myforest. 32(1), pp53-58. 1987

Ndiaye, B.S. and A. Sene. (In French) Rapport de l'Evaluation du Projet Test de Lutte Contre la Malnutrition a Base des Produits du *Moringa oleifera* dans la Region de Zigguinchor. (Unpublished document). 1998

Nwosu, M.O., and J.I. Okafor. "Preliminary studies of the antifungal activities of some medicinal plants against *Basidiobolus* and some other pathological fungi". Mycoses. 38, pp. 191-195. 1995

Pal, S.K., P.K. Mukherjee and B.P. Saha. "Studies on the antiulcer activity of *Moringa oleifera* leaf extract on gastric ulcer models in rats". Phytotherapy Research. 9, pp 463-465. 1995

Pal, S.K., P.K. Mukherjee, K. Saha, M. Pal and B.P. Saha. "Studies on some psychopharmacalogical actions of *Moringa oleifera* Lam. (Moringaceae) leaf extract". Phytotherapy Research. 10, pp. 402-405. 1996

Palada, M.C. "Moringa (*Moringa oleifera* Lam.): A versitile tree crop with horticultural potential in the subtropical United States". HortScience. 31(5), September 1996

Quisumbing, E. *Moringa oleifera* Lam., Medicinal Plants of the Philippines. Katha Publications. pp. 346-349. 1978

Ram, J. Moringa a highly nutritious vegetable tree. Technical Bulletin No. 2. Tropical Rural and Island/Atoll Development Experimental Station (TRIADES). 1994

Ramachandran, C., K.V. Peter and P.K. Gopalakrishnan. "Drumstick (*Moringa oleifera*): A multipurpose Indian vegetable". Economic Botany. 34(3), pp 276-283. 1980

Rao Kurma, S., and S.H. Mishra. "Drumstick polysaccharide as pharmaceutical adjuvant". Indian Journal of Natural Products. 9(1), pp 3-6. 1993

Saint Sauveur, A. (In French) Le *Moringa oleifera* au Niger et en Inde, ou Quand les Agriculteurs Preferment Planter les Arbres. Le Flamboyant, Silva. 43, pp. 16-23. September 1997

Scrimshaw, N. and R. Morgan. Improving the Nutritional Status of Children During the Weaning Period. FAO/WHO/UNU. 1983

Subadra, S., J. Monica and D. Dhabhai. "Retention and storage stability of beta-carotene in dehydrated drumstick leaves (*Moringa oleifera*)". International Journal of Food Sciences and Nutrition. 48, pp. 373-379. 1997

Sunga, I. and G. Whitby. "Decentralized edible oil milling in Zimbabwe: an evaluation report of the Tinytech oil mill project". Progress Report for Intermediate Technology Development Group. Rugby, UK. 1995

Sutherland, J.P., G.K. Folkard and W.D. Grant. "Natural coagulants for appropriate water treatment: a novel approach". Waterlines. April, 8(4), pp 30-32. 1990

Sutherland, J.P., G.K. Folkard, M.A. Mtawali and W.D. Grant. "*Moringa oleifera* at pilot/full scale". In: J. Pickford et al eds. Water, Sanitation, Environment and Development: Proceedings of the 19th WEDC Conference, Accra, Ghana, September 1993. Loughborough University of Technology Press. pp 109-111. 1994

Tauscher, B. "Water treatment by flocculant compounds of higher plants". Plant Research and Development. 40, pp 56-70. 1994

Udupa, S.L. A.l. Udupa and D.R. Kulkarni. "Studies on the anti-inflammatory and wound healing properties of *Moringa oleifera* and *Aegle marmelos*". Fitoterapia. 65(2), pp 119-123. 1994

Verdcourt, B. "A synopsis of the Moringaceae". Kew Bulletin. 40(1), pp 1-34. 1985

Verma, S.C., R. Banerji, G. Misra, S.K. Nigum "Nutritional value of Moringa". Current Science. 45(21), pp 769-770

Vietmeyer, N. "New crops: Solutions for global problems". pp. 2-8. In: J. Janick (ed.), Progress in New Crops. ASHS Press. Alexandria, Virginia. 1996

Von Maydell, H.J. Trees and Shrubs of the Sahel, Their Characteristics and Uses. Pub: GTZ, Eschborn, Germany. 1986

Watson, L., and M.J. Dallwitz The Families of Flowering Plants. Published online only, at http://biodiversity.uno.edu/delta. 1992 onwards; version: 19th August 1999.

Index

Holism and Evolution

The concept and word "holistic" were created in this classic book in 1926...now available in a new edition

The growing popularity of holistic health and a more natural way of living is only the first of many ways this thoughtful approach to life is changing the world we live in.

Much of the attractiveness of holistic health and the natural life can be traced to the sympathetic chord they have struck with millions of people seeking a more balanced life. But this did not happen by accident. As you will see, the holistic approach to life is so deeply in tune with everything that happens in the world around us that it naturally stirs something profound and satisfying within us.

Holism and Evolution is available through bookstores and other retail sources. If you do not find it there, it can be mailed to you.

(Use order form on the next page)

Have your own copy of

Holism and Evolution

Or send one to a friend

It's as easy as . . .

1. Tell us where to send it:

Name_____

Address_____

City_____State____Zip_____

If it's a gift, fill in your name:

It's a gift from

_____

2. And send a check or money order for

Book 24.95
Shipping 2.95
$ 27.90

California residents add sales
tax for a total of **$ 29.90**

Library
Quality
Hardcover
Book

3. To: Sierra Sunrise Books
14622 Ventura Blvd, # 800
Sherman Oaks, CA 91403

(Allow 2-4 weeks for delivery)
(You may copy this order form)

Mor-1

Books by Sanford Holst (author)

LifeCycle

What do you want most in life? The guidelines in *LifeCycle* put you quickly on the best path to get there.

Beginning with insights on where you are today, you're soon exploring the essential parts of your life and the natural connections between them. That new understanding gives you a significant advantage in getting what you want and need.

You can enjoy all five parts of a complete and satisfying life: healthy body, great relationships, successful career, enjoyable surroundings and peace of mind.

The connections between these key parts of your life multiply the benefit of each step you take. After a few small steps, your life is remarkably better. And as you continue, the benefits multiply even more.

Whatever you want most is waiting for you.

LifeCycle is available through bookstores and other retail sources. If you do not find it there, it can be mailed to you.

(Use order form on next page)

Have your own copy of

LifeCycle

Or send one to a friend

It's as easy as . . .

1. Tell us where to send it:

Name_____

Address_____

City_____State_____Zip_____

If it's a gift, fill in your name:

It's a gift from

_____

2. And send a check or money order for

Book 18.95
Shipping 2.40
$ 21.35

California residents add sales
tax for a total of **$ 22.95**

Library
Quality
Hardcover
Book

3. To: Sierra Sunrise Books
14622 Ventura Blvd, # 800
Sherman Oaks, CA 91403

(Allow 2-4 weeks for delivery)
(You may copy this order form)

Mor-1

Moringa

*M*oringa: **Nature's Medicine Cabinet** is available through bookstores and other retail sources. If for any reason you do not find it there, you can order a copy and have it mailed to you.

(Use order form on the next page)

Have your own copy of

Moringa

Or send one to a friend

It's as easy as . . .

1. Tell us where to send it:

Name_____

Address_____

City_____State____Zip_____

If it's a gift, fill in your name:

It's a gift from

_____

2. And send a check or money order for

Book 9.95

Shipping . . . .   <u>1.95</u>

$ 11.90

California residents add sales
tax for a total of **$ 12.90**

3. To: Sierra Sunrise Books
14622 Ventura Blvd, # 800
Sherman Oaks, CA 91403

(Allow 2-4 weeks for delivery)
(You may copy this order form)   Mor-1